The AAMT Book of Style

Student Workbook:
Practical Application and Assessment

American Association for Medical Transcription

The AAMT Book of Style

Student Workbook:
Practical Application and Assessment

American Association for Medical Transcription
Lea M. Sims, CMT, FAAMT

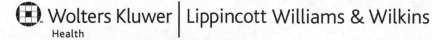

Wolters Kluwer | Lippincott Williams & Wilkins
Health

Philadelphia · Baltimore · New York · London
Buenos Aires · Hong Kong · Sydney · Tokyo

Publisher: Julie Stegman
Senior Product Manager: Eric Branger
Managing Editor: Amy Millholen
Copyeditor: Diane Heath
Proofreader: Kristin Wall
Marketing Manager: Chris Kushner
Interior Design: Lou Fuiano, Fuiano Design
Cover Design: Jason Delaney
Compositor: Maryland Composition
Printer: RR Donnelley

DISCLAIMER

Care has been taken to confirm the accuracy of the information present and to describe generally accepted practices. However, the authors, editors, and publisher are not responsible for errors
or omissions or for any consequences from application of the information in this book and make
no warranty, expressed or implied, with respect to the currency, completeness, or accuracy of the
contents of the publication. Application of this information in a particular situation remains the
professional responsibility of the practitioner; the clinical treatments described and recommended
may not be considered absolute and universal recommendations.

ISBN 0-7817-6001-1

Printed in the United States of America

To purchase additional copies of this book, call our customer service department at (800) 638-3030
or fax orders to (301) 824-7390. For other book services, including chapter reprints and large quantity sales, ask for the Special Sales department.

For all other calls originating outside of the United States, please call (301) 714-2324.

Visit Lippincott Williams & Wilkins on the Internet: http://www.lww.com. Lippincott Williams
& Wilkins customer service representatives are available from 8:30 am to 6:00 pm, EST, Monday
through Friday, for telephone access.

07 08 09
1 2 3 4 5 6 7 8 9 10

Dedication

For every MT with an eye for detail
Who believes that a standard should always prevail
Who takes extra minutes to make it "just so"
And knows where all pesky commas should go
Who seeks to know always just what to do,
This Book of Style Workbook is written for *you*.

And if you're an MT who just hasn't a clue,
Well…this workbook is written just for *you, too*.

- Lea M. Sims, CMT, FAAMT

Preface

Since its original publication, *The AAMT Book of Style (BOS)* has become the recognized industry resource for medical transcription style and standards. It is widely utilized in the corporate and institutional setting.

An MT's understanding and successful application of these standards of practice is critical to future and ongoing quality assessment in the marketplace. The industry has placed a high value on quality and the application of tools and assessments to evaluate that level of quality for its practitioners. In 2004, AAMT released its position on Quality Assurance for Medical Transcription, urging employers in the industry to institute measurable assessments for ongoing quality assurance, citing the dynamic impact quality documentation has on continuity of patient care, risk management, and reimbursement. To that end, the position paper further urges the industry to embrace the standards outlined in the *Book of Style* in both its training and quality assurance measures. Industry surveys have indicated a strong preference in the institutional and corporate sectors for the standards outlined in the *BOS* when establishing training programs and ongoing QA policies.

The need to respond to this industry dynamic is continually addressed at the educational level when developing degree programs and vocational technical programs for medical transcription. Educational institutions and programs have recognized the industry demand for MTs who are trained and familiar with *The AAMT Book of Style* and have included it in their curricula as well as adopted the book as required text in the classroom. However, the dilemma for instructors hoping to incorporate standards into their established course outline still remains. How can this obviously essential book of industry standards be effectively utilized in a classroom setting when it was clearly not designed to be used in this way? In essence, how does one teach from a dictionary-style text?

Feedback to AAMT via educator's conferences and other surveys has indicated an undeniable need in the education and training setting for a companion manual to the current *BOS*, one that addresses the standards in a topical and organized fashion and provides opportunity for review, self-assessment, and in-class testing of same.

In response, Lea Sims, CMT, FAAMT, Director of Communications for AAMT, has written a workbook with a unit/chapter organizational approach to accompany *The AAMT Book of Style* in the classroom and in the corporate setting where formal and informal continuing education is carried out. This *Workbook* will serve to instruct in the application of standards as well as prepare, review, and test students and practitioners in the field who will sit for the national certification exam.

Organization

As a reference tool, the *BOS* is appropriately organized as an alphabetical index of concepts and topics, related to present trends and practices in the industry, whose prevalent application and usage have necessitated their inclusion.

In this *Workbook*, however, the author has used a topical and unit approach, pulling together the most significant and essential standards of style, grouping them first by topics and then by unit. The *Workbook* is divided into six units and 20 chapters. For example, Unit 1, Abbreviations, Acronyms & Brief Forms, contains three chapters—Abbreviations and Acronyms: Rules and Exceptions; Dangerous Abbreviations; and Acceptable Forms, Back Formations & Slang. Unit 5 organizes those standards specifically related to specialties into four separate chapters. Unit 6, the final unit, pulls those standards less easily classified into three separate chapters.

For each topic, the current standard provided in the *BOS* is succinctly restated, and a quick reference to the relevant section in the *BOS* is provided. In "Going Deeper," additional explanation is provided to ensure understanding and to promote memorization of standards that simply cannot be learned by any other method. Since many of these standards incorporate grammar rules, conceptual understanding alone will not carry a student to consistency. There are many areas that quite simply must be first memorized, then understood, and then evaluated. The concepts addressed in this manual are elementary, but many will introduce information that would not have been encountered outside of healthcare documentation and will therefore be completely unknown to the student. Additional features to aid learning and memorization include the addition of application examples and boxes to highlight important concepts.

While this *Workbook* does expand on the current *BOS* in terms of more detailed explanations and examples, there are no new or "cutting edge" concepts introduced. The primary purpose of this text is to provide a better organization of *BOS* topics for classroom use, not to introduce new material.

Ancillary Resources

Perhaps the most outstanding feature of this package, other than the organizational approach to teaching concepts not previously available in this format, is the CD-ROM containing dictation clips that may be used for additional practice in applying the standards being studied, self-assessment, or for testing purposes. The Appendices to accompany the *Workbook* are on the CD-ROM, as well. Additional dictation tests are provided in the *Instructor's Manual*, which is posted in the Instructors section of the companion website for the *Workbook*. The Student section of the website includes the Appendices for the *Workbook*, and also includes the dictation practice exercises. To access the online student and instructor resources, go to http://thePoint.lww.com/aamtstudent.

Prior to this time, attempts to test students in the area of style application have been entirely in written format, which is limited in its ability to provide a truly realistic transcription simulation. The very nature of a written question implies that it has been removed from the interpretive role necessary to transcription. Having dictated questions for review and testing will produce a more realistic training environment for the MT, who has to rely on auditory interpretation for application of standards without the help of "suggestion" inherently provided in a written question.

This *Workbook* was written and designed primarily for students in MT education programs—community college AS-degree programs, technical or vocational credit programs, vocational schools, and online MT programs. However, it lends itself well to other settings as well as independent study. National MT companies who have instituted full-fledged on-site training programs will want to adopt it as well. The *Workbook* should be just as useful for new hires and continuing education for MT practitioners in all settings. In addition, anyone preparing to take the CMT examination will find the organization of this *Workbook* and the self-assessment materials beneficial in preparation for those aspects of the exam that will address *Book of Style* standards.

There are other grammar and punctuation, as well as transcription skills workbooks, available in the industry. Many educators utilize them as the only option available to them in addressing the practical application issues in transcription training that fall outside the scope of anatomy, medical terminology, or healthcare knowledge. However, there is no workbook that stems directly from the industry standard manual, which is *The AAMT Book of Style*. There are some workbooks out there that cite the *BOS* as a "reference" or claim to "follow" the *BOS*, but none that are endorsed by AAMT and designed to actually *teach* this industry-recognized reference—until now.

The AAMT Book of Style Workbook combined with *The AAMT Book of Style* makes an ideal text for a medical grammar and style course in an MT program. This *Workbook* answers a need that has existed since the publication of the original *AAMT Book of Style*. No medical transcription education program should be without it.

Ellen Drake, CMT, FAAMT

Acknowledgements

Projects of this magnitude are always a beautiful collaboration, and this one was no exception. I am very grateful for the input and wisdom of many who have contributed to this much-needed text for medical transcription students.

I would like to acknowledge first and foremost the visionary thinking of Claudia Tessier, RHIA, CAE, and Sally C. Pitman, who along with their colleagues first conceived of a resource for medical transcription standards for style. That early collaboration became the "gold" standard that paved the way for future editions of the current *AAMT Book of Style*. Peg Hughes, CMT, Diane Heath, CMT, and Kathy Rockel, CMT, FAAMT, assumed the mantle of updating that text to the 2nd edition in circulation today. It is that research and content development that enabled the *Student Workbook* you are now reading. Thank you to those fine professionals for laying a solid foundation that made my job here so much easier.

A supportive network of industry colleagues and content experts is essential to any author or editor. I was fortunate to have some incredible minds at my disposal. Ellen Drake, CMT, FAAMT; Laura Bryan, CMT, FAAMT; Diana Gish, CMT, FAAMT; and Kristin Wall have been an invaluable source of support and feedback through this process. I also want to thank Peter Preziosi, PhD, CAE – not only a supportive employer who empowers me to succeed but also a true friend.

Thank you to Stedman's for an amazing working relationship and your patience as I slowly plugged away at this project in the midst of other responsibilities and commitments. You truly are a blessed resource for our industry.

Finally, I want to thank my husband, Grady, and my children, Peyton and Madison, for their love, support, and understanding when Mom's hours at the computer were seemingly unending. You make it all worthwhile.

Lea M. Sims, CMT, FAAMT

Reviewers

The publisher and author gratefully acknowledge the professionals who served as reviewers of this textbook. These individuals include:

Diana Gish, CMT, FAAMT
AAMT Staff, Educational Approval
M-TEC, Instructor
MedQuist, Quality Specialist
Phoenix, AZ

Carolyn Grimes, MS, CMT, RHIA, FAAMT
Instructor
M-TEC
Homestead, FL

Diane S. Heath, CMT
MT Project Consultant
Dallas, TX

Sandra King, RN, CMT, FAAMT
QA Mentor/Educator
Webmedx
Charlotte, MI

Janice Tatrow, BSBA, AAS
Adjunct Faculty, Health & Information Technology
Davenport University
Holland, MI

Table of Contents

Abbreviations, Acronyms & Brief Forms

1

Abbreviations and Acronyms
Rules and Exceptions

BOS Statement

Where?
BOS pp. 1–3

Abbreviations, acronyms, and brief forms are often used in medical dictation to speed up communication, but they frequently create confusion instead. While the originator may think that dictating the abbreviation *AML* is the fastest way to communicate *acute myelocytic leukemia*, medical transcriptionists know better. They face the dilemma: Does *AML* mean acute monocytic leukemia, acute myeloblastic leukemia, acute myelocytic leukemia, acute myelogenous leukemia, acute myeloid leukemia, or perhaps even some less common alternative? In the numerous publications devoted to translating medical abbreviations, abbreviations with single meaning appear to be in the minority.

Clarity of communication is essential. Avoid the use of abbreviations, acronyms, and brief forms except for internationally recognized and accepted units of measure and for widely recognized terms and symbols. Do not use any that readers will not immediately recognize. Unless the abbreviation, acronym, or brief form is so widely used that it has in essence become a term in its own right, use the expanded form first, followed by its abbreviated form in parentheses. Then use the abbreviated form throughout the remainder of the document.

There is no nationally recognized list of approved abbreviations for use in medical reports, nor does AAMT propose such a list. However, it is important to note that the Joint Commission on Accreditation of Healthcare Organizations (JCAHO) requires that in order to be accredited a hospital should use uniform data definitions whenever possible; they note that an abbreviation list (which might be interpreted as a list of abbreviations to avoid) is one way to meet this requirement.

Going Deeper

The use of abbreviations in health encounter documentation is widely prevalent. There are many factors and considerations that have to be taken into account when establishing practices and policies governing their use in transcription. As outlined above from the BOS, the primary consideration for the expansion or retention of a dictated abbreviation should be the promotion of clarity. Attention must be paid to the potential for misinterpretation when encountering abbreviations in dictation. However, it is important to note that there are other potential considerations that an MT will ultimately encounter in the workplace.

Facility Policy   As with other points of style and standards, provider/client preference will often be the final word on this issue. A healthcare provider or facility that is concerned about transcription costs, particularly in a per-unit billing environment, may restrict the expansion of many abbreviations despite the standards outlined here. Other providers and facilities may be more risk-management-minded and may require the expansion of all abbreviations. It is important for the MT student to be aware that variability in the application of these standards may exist in the job setting.

Productivity   It is important to note that the decision to expand an abbreviation should never be made on the basis of its impact on productivity or potential wages, even in the absence of a company policy or provider preference. Transcribing a dictated abbreviation in abbreviated or expanded form should be based on the rules and exceptions outlined in this text with consideration for facility policies. The utilization of word-expansion software to increase productivity often facilitates the quick and easy expansion of any and all abbreviations encountered in dictation; however, their expansion or retention should be judiciously considered on the basis of these principles and not on productivity goals.

This chapter outlines the rules and exceptions related to abbreviations and acronyms, beginning with fundamental definitions.

Definitions

Abbreviation A shortened form of a word or phrase used chiefly in writing, such as *USMC* for *United States Marine Corps*. **Types:** Acronyms, initialisms, and brief forms

Acronym An abbreviation formed from the initial letters of each of the successive words or major parts of a compound term or of selected letters of a word or phrase **that is pronounced as a word** (e.g., *AIDS, GERD,* and *LASIK*).

Initialism An abbreviation formed from the initial letters of each of the successive words or major parts of a compound term or of selected letters of a word or phrase **that is not pronounced as a word but by each letter** (e.g., *ALS, CPK,* and *HIV*).

Brief Forms An abbreviation that results in a shortened form of a single word rather than the initial letters of a series of words (e.g., *phone, exam, Pap smear,* and *labs*). See Chapter 3 for more information about brief forms.

Rules & Exceptions

I. When and Why | Transcribe abbreviations if they are commonly used and widely recognized. Again, clarity is the goal in making these transcription decisions. Remember the following rules and exceptions:

A   **Terms dictated in full.** Do not use an abbreviation when a term is dictated in full.

Exception: Units of measure (milligrams, centimeters, etc.).

B   **Diagnosis and operative titles.** Write out an abbreviation in full if it is used in the admission, discharge, preoperative, or postoperative diagnosis; consultative conclusion; or operative title. These are critical points of information, and their meanings must be clear to ensure accurate communication for patient care, reimbursement, statistical purposes, and medicolegal documentation.

> DICTATED
> **DIAGNOSIS: CAD.**
>
> TRANSCRIBED
> **DIAGNOSIS: Coronary artery disease (CAD).**

Exceptions: 1. Non-disease-entity abbreviations (laboratory tests, units of measure, etc.). When these accompany diagnostic and procedure statements, they may be used if dictated. **2.** Abbreviations best known abbreviated (HIV, AIDS, etc.). Some disease entities are better-known and widely referred to by their abbreviated forms, and to expand them would actually make the meaning less clear. In those rare instances, retain the abbreviation no matter where in the report that reference occurs.

C   **Multiple or uncertain meanings.** When an abbreviated diagnosis, conclusion, or operative title is dictated and the abbreviation used is not familiar or has multiple meanings, the meaning may be discerned if the originator uses the extended term elsewhere in the dictation or if the content of the report somehow makes the meaning obvious. If the extended form cannot be determined in this way and there is easy and immediate access to the patient's record or to the person who dictated the report, the MT should use these as resources to determine the meaning. If these attempts are unsuccessful, the abbreviated form should be transcribed as dictated and then flagged with a request for the originator to provide the extended form.

> DICTATED
> **DIAGNOSIS: AML.**
>
> TRANSCRIBED
> **DIAGNOSIS: AML.**
>
> *Flag report for verification.*

D

Units of measure.

1. Abbreviate most *metric* units of measure that accompany numerals and include virgule constructions. Use the same abbreviation for singular and plural forms. Do not use periods with abbreviated units of measure. Use these abbreviations only when a numeric quantity precedes the unit of measure.

> **She was put on 2 L of oxygen.**
> **An approximately 2.5 cm incision was made.**
>
> *but*
>
> **The wound measured several centimeters.**

2. Spell out common *nonmetric* units of measure to express weight, depth, distance, height, length, and width, except in tables. Do not abbreviate most nonmetric units of measure, except in tables.

> **The baby weighed 8 pounds 9 ounces.**
> **She gave the child 2 tablespoons of Motrin.**

E

Dangerous and obscure abbreviations. Do not use abbreviations found on the "Dangerous Abbreviations" list from the Institute for Safe Medication Practices (see Chapter 2). In addition to those found on the list, avoid any abbreviation that is obscure (like *a.c.b.* for "before breakfast") or any others that are potentially dangerous. For example, *b.i.w.* is both obscure and dangerous. It is intended to mean *twice weekly*, but it could be mistaken for *twice daily*, resulting in a dosage frequency seven times that intended.

F

Business names. Some businesses are readily recognized by their abbreviations or acronyms and may be referred to by the same if dictated and if there is reasonable assurance the business will be accurately identified by the reader. Most abbreviated forms use all capitals and do not use periods, but be guided by the entity's designated abbreviated form.

> **IBM equipment**
> **He is an ACLU attorney.**
> **She found the item on eBay.**

G

Geographic names. Abbreviate state and territory names when they are preceded by a city, state or territory name. Do not abbreviate names of states, territories, countries or similar units within reports when they stand alone. Use abbreviations in state names in an address (such as in a letter or on an envelope).

> **She was seen in an ER in Orlando, FL, a month ago.**
> **The patient moved here 3 years ago from Canada.**

H

Units of time. Do not abbreviate English units of time except in virgule (slash) constructions. Do not use periods with such abbreviations.

> **The patient is 5 days old.**
> **He will return in 1 week for followup.**
> **Her IV was set to run at 10 mcg/min while in the ER.**

I

Slang, jargon, and coined terms. Due to the evolutionary nature of our language, clinicians sometimes find themselves dictating in clipped terms to expedite their documentation. The result may be awkward, poorly cast brief forms that need to be expanded for clarity. Be sure to consult an abbreviations and acronyms resource book to determine which abbreviations are considered slang and should be expanded.

> DICTATED
> **Stool was guaiac'd.**
>
> TRANSCRIBED
> **Stool guaiac test was done.**

DICTATED
She had an appy at age 22.

TRANSCRIBED
She had an appendectomy at age 22.

DICTATED
The vessels were bovied and hemostasis was achieved.

TRANSCRIBED
The vessels were cauterized with a Bovie, and hemostasis was achieved.

II. Grammar and Punctuation

A   **Placement.**
1. A sentence may begin with a dictated abbreviation, or such abbreviated forms may be expanded.

DICTATED
WBC was 9200.

TRANSCRIBED
WBC was 9200.

or

White blood count was 9200.

2. Avoid separating a numeral from its associated unit of measure or accompanying abbreviation; that is, keep the numeral and unit of measure together at line breaks.

. . . .**The specimen measured 4 cm in diameter.**
or

. . . .**The specimen measured 4 cm in diameter.**

> *not*
>
> . . . . .The specimen measured 4
> cm in diameter.

B   **Capitalization.**
1. Capitalize all letters of most acronyms, but when they are expanded, do not capitalize the words from which they are formed unless they are proper names.

> **AIDS (<u>a</u>cquired <u>i</u>mmuno<u>d</u>eficiency <u>s</u>yndrome)**
> **BiPAP (<u>b</u>ilateral <u>p</u>ositive <u>a</u>irway <u>p</u>ressure)**
> **TURP (<u>t</u>rans<u>u</u>rethral <u>r</u>esection of <u>p</u>rostate)**

2. Do not capitalize abbreviations derived from Latin terms. The use of periods within or at the end of these Latin abbreviations remains the preferred style, although it is also acceptable to drop the periods for general Latin terms.

Use lowercase abbreviations with periods for Latin abbreviations that are related to doses and dosages. Avoid using all capitals because they emphasize the abbreviation rather than the drug name. Avoid lower-case abbreviations without periods because some may be misread as words.

> | **e.g.** | *exempli gratia* | **for example** |
> |---|---|---|
> | **et al.** | *et alii* | **and others** |
> | **etc.** | *et cetera* | **and so forth** |
> | **a.c.** | *ante cibum* | **before food** |
> | **b.i.d.** | *bis in die* | **twice a day** |

3. Do not capitalize a brief form unless the extended form is routinely capitalized.

> | **segmented neutrophils** | **segs** |
> |---|---|
> | **examination** | **exam** |
> | **Papanicolaou smear** | **Pap smear** |
> | **Kirschner wire** | **K-wire** |

4. Do not capitalize most units of measure or their abbreviations. Learn the obvious exceptions, and consult appropriate references for guidance.

EXAMPLES			
meter	m	kilogram	kg
mole	mol	centimeter	cm

EXCEPTIONS			
liter	L	kelvin	K
milliliter	mL	ampere	A
decibel	dB	hertz	Hz
joule	J	milliequivalent	mEq

5. Always capitalize genus name abbreviations when they are accompanied by the species name.

H influenzae
E coli
C difficile

C **Punctuation.**
1. Do not use periods within or at the end of most abbreviations, including acronyms, abbreviated units of measure, and brief forms. Use a period at the end of abbreviated English units of measure if they may be misread without the period (only in virgule constructions and tables).

wbc	WBC	mg	cm
exam	prep	mEq	mL

inch preferred to *in*.
(Do not use *in* for *inch* without a period)

2. Do not use periods with abbreviated academic degrees and professional credentials.

John Smith, MD
Mary Jones, CMT
Robert Williams, PhD

3. Use periods in lowercase drug-related abbreviations derived from Latin terms.

b.i.d.	**t.i.d.**	**a.c.**
p.r.n.	**p.o.**	**q.4 h.**

NOTE: AAMT continues to discourage dropping periods in lowercase abbreviations that might be misread as words (bid and tid). If you must drop the periods, use all capitals, but keep in mind that the overuse of capitals, particularly in relation to drug doses and dosages, would draw more attention to the capitalized abbreviations than to the drug names themselves.

4. Periods may be used with courtesy title abbreviations (e.g., Mr., Mrs.) and following Jr. and Sr., although there is a trend toward dropping them; either remains acceptable, but be consistent.

5. Use a lowercase *s* without an apostrophe to form the plural of a capitalized abbreviation, acronym, or brief form.

EKGs	**PVCs**	**exams**
labs	**monos**	**CABGs**

6. Use *'s* to form the plural of lowercase abbreviations.

rbc's	**wbc's**

7. Use *'s* to form the plural of single-letter abbreviations.

X's	**K's**	**flipped T's**

8. Add *'s* to most abbreviations or acronyms to show possession.

The AMA's address is...
AAMT's position paper on full disclosure states...

The Final Word

Ultimately, the application of these standards comes down to some fundamental common-sense principles. The objective, as stated initially, is to promote clarity in the healthcare record. An abbreviated form, when used, should meet this objective, and the application of capitalization or the use of punctuation to indicate plurality or possession should likewise promote clarity and be used consistently throughout the healthcare record. Of course, the overall goal of these standards is to encourage their consistent use across the entire healthcare delivery system.

QUICK REVIEW

1. Use dictated abbreviations in all areas of the report except the diagnosis and operative title sections if the abbreviation promotes clarity, is widely recognized, and could not be misinterpreted.

2. Do not abbreviate terms dictated in full except for units of measure.

3. Abbreviate metric units of measure. Do not abbreviate nonmetric units of measure.

4. Do not use abbreviations found on the "Dangerous Abbreviations" list (see Chapter 2).

5. Abbreviate business names if that is the entity's preference.

6. Abbreviate state names when preceded by a city. Spell them out when they occur alone in the sentence. Use abbreviations in state names in an address (such as in a letter or on an envelope).

7. Do not abbreviate English units of time.

8. Abbreviations can be used at the beginning of the sentence.

9. Unit-of-measure abbreviations that wrap to a second line should be adjusted to accompany the value that precedes or follows them.

10. Capitalize initialisms and acronyms by consulting industry references.

11. Do not capitalize abbreviations formed from Latin terms.

12. Capitalize brief forms only if the extended form is capitalized.

13. Be aware of and learn which unit-of-measure abbreviations are lowercased and which are capitalized.

14. Capitalize genus name abbreviations when accompanied by the species name.

15. Do not use periods within or at the end of any abbreviation unless it is an abbreviation derived from a Latin term.

16. Add an *s* to form the plural of capitalized abbreviations and acronyms. Add an *s* to form the plural of a brief form.

17. Add an *'s* to form the plural of lowercased abbreviations and single letters.

18. Add an *'s* to most abbreviations and acronyms to show possession.

Test Your Knowledge

Select the correct answer from the options provided below each question. Record the letter corresponding to your answer on the line provided.

_____ 1. **Which of the following is an example of an ACRONYM?**
A. COPD
B. t.i.d.
C. CABG
D. lymphs

_____ 2. **Which of the following is an example of a BRIEF FORM?**
A. cath
B. mmHg
C. BKA
D. All of the above

_____ 3. **Which is correctly transcribed?**
A. TITLE OF OPERATION: ORIF, left radius.
B. DIAGNOSIS: Pyelonephritis with elevated blood urea nitrogen (BUN).
C. TITLE OF OPERATION: Transurethral resection of the prostate (TURP).
D. DIAGNOSIS: IDDM.

_____ 4. **A measurement would be correctly indicated by which of the following?**
A. 2 cm
B. 3 inches
C. a few centimeters
D. All of the above

_____ 5. **Which would represent the incorrect transcription of a measurement?**
A. 4.5 cm
B. 3 in
C. 4 feet
D. All of the above.

_____ 6. The Latin abbreviation meaning "twice per day" would be correctly transcribed as:
A. bid
B. B.I.D.
C. b.i.d.
D. BID

_____ 7. Which represents the incorrect capitalization of an abbreviation?
A. Differential showed 58 SEGs.
B. WBC was 48.2.
C. Urinalysis revealed 8-10 wbc's.
D. None of the above

_____ 8. Which of the following is correctly pluralized?
A. serial K's
B. EKG's
C. lymph's
D. rbcs

_____ 9. Which of the following genus/species references is correctly transcribed?
A. staphylococcus aureus
B. s. aureus
C. S Aureus
D. S aureus

_____ 10. Which of the following is correctly transcribed?
A. The baby weighed 8 lbs 12 oz.
B. She was instructed to return on a prn basis.
C. We injected 10 mL of lidocaine.
D. CBC showed WBC's of 9.2.

Test Your Knowledge

Answers

1. C

2. A

3. C

4. D

5. B

6. C

7. A

8. A

9. D

10. C

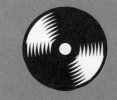

APPLICATION TEST
Take the application test for this chapter on your CD-ROM.
Access the section for
Chapter 1: "Abbreviations and Acronyms."

Dangerous Abbreviations

BOS Statement

Where?
BOS p. 2

Some abbreviations, particularly with respect to medication orders, have proven to be dangerous. For example, the *U* in *insulin 6 U* could possibly be misread as a zero, or a medication that is given once a day may mistakenly be given four times a day if *q.d.* were misread as *q.i.d.* These types of errors can and do happen and have at times caused fatalities.

Organizations involved in identifying and preventing such problems include the United States Pharmacopeia (USP), the Institute for Safe Medication Practices (ISMP), the US Food and Drug Administration (FDA), and the National Coordinating Council for Medication Error Reporting and Prevention (NCC MERP). ISMP has published a list of dangerous abbreviations and dose designations as reported to the USP-ISMP Medication Errors Reporting Program, and AAMT has chosen to promote the adoption of this list.

Going Deeper

Almost 50% of the Joint Commission on Accreditation of Healthcare Organizations (JCAHO) standards is directly related to patient safety in some way. In July of 2002, the Joint Commission approved its first six (6) National Patient Safety Goals (NPSGs), designed to improve safety measures in identified key areas of patient management and care. In 2004, the Joint Commission began developing program-specific NPSGs for each of its accreditation and certification programs. Goal 2, "Improve the effectiveness of communication among caregivers," speaks specifically to the quality of communication among members of the healthcare team.

The second directive of Goal 2 addresses the subject of abbreviations: "Standardize a list of abbreviations, acronyms and symbols that are *not* to be used throughout the organization."

This directive generated quite a response from the healthcare community, because JCAHO included as part of this goal a list of abbreviations considered so dangerous that their use would be prohibited in the healthcare setting and would be part of future standards by which healthcare organizations would be measured. The original list recommended by the ISMP, found on page 461 of *The AAMT Book of Style for Medical Transcription*, 2nd edition, and delineated later in this chapter, was quite extensive. The prospect of changing and/or upgrading pharmaceutical processes, programs, and software systems to reflect these new abbreviation standards has been daunting, and the cost associated with those changes has in many cases been prohibitive. According to the Joint Commission's NPSG website frequently asked questions list:

The long-term objective of this requirement continues to be 100 percent compliance, in all forms of clinical documentation, with a reasonably comprehensive list of prohibited "dangerous" abbreviations, acronyms and symbols. However, recognizing that this type of change will take time, the survey and scoring of this requirement has been modified, effective immediately, for surveys conducted through the end of 2004, as follows:

If, on survey, the organization has not yet achieved 100 percent compliance as evidenced by open and closed medical record review, a score of "In compliance" will be recorded if the following conditions are met:

- *Use of any item on the list is "sporadic" (less than 10 percent of the instances of the intended term are abbreviated or symbolized); AND*
- *Whenever any prohibited item has been used in an order, there is written evidence of confirmation of the intended meaning before the order is carried out; AND*
- *The organization has implemented a plan for continued improvement to achieve 100 percent compliance by the end of 2004.*

In other words, the Joint Commission is allowing for the fact that transition to this new standard will take time. A facility will have to demonstrate that it has made reasonable efforts to ensure that the abbreviations on the "do not use" list have been eliminated from all patient care documentation as the facility transitions to full compliance.

As a transcriptionist in that environment, it will be important to understand the evolution of this standard and how strictly it may be applied by your employer. While you are still in the early learning stages of this new career, it is best to spend time learning and memorizing all of the abbreviations considered to be dangerous and editing those abbreviations appropriately when you encounter them in dictation since, out of habit, many dictators will still continue to use those abbreviations.

Rules & Exceptions

JCAHO "Dangerous Abbreviations" List

Given the fact that transition to a full and comprehensive list of dangerous abbreviations, such as those outlined in the BOS, has been deemed to be unreasonable in the short term, the Joint Commission has released a "minimum list" of abbreviations that "must be included on each accredited organization's 'do not use' list." These are as follows:

Set	Item	Abbreviation	Potential Problem	Preferred Term
1.	1.	U (for unit)	Mistaken as zero, four, or cc	Write "unit"
2.	2.	IU (for international unit)	Mistaken as IV (intravenous) or 10 (ten)	Write "international unit"
3.	3. 4.	q.d. or Q.D. q.o.d. or Q.O.D. (Latin abbreviation for once daily and every other day)	Mistaken for each . other. The period after the *Q* can be mistaken for an *I* and the *O* can be mistaken for *I*	Write "daily" and "every other day"
4.	5. 6.	Trailing zero (X.0 mg) [Note: Prohibited only for medication-related notations]; Lack of leading zero (.X mg)	Decimal point is missed	Never write a zero by itself after a decimal point (X mg), and always use a zero before a decimal point (0.X mg)

5.	7.	MS	Confused for one	Write "morphine
	8.	MSO4	another	sulfate" or
	9.	MgSO4	Can mean morphine	"magnesium
			sulfate or magnesium	sulfate"
			sulfate	

In addition to this minimum list, JCAHO required any organization that did not already have a banned list of abbreviations in place to identify and apply at least another 3 "do not use" abbreviations, acronyms, or symbols of its choosing (effective April 1, 2004). JCAHO recommends selecting those additional "do not use" items from the following list of additional abbreviations considered to be dangerous:

µg (for microgram)	Mistaken for mg (milligrams) resulting in one thousand-fold dosing overdose	Write "mcg"
h.s. or H.S. (for half-strength or Latin abbreviation for bedtime)	Mistaken for either half-strength or hour of sleep (at bedtime). Likewise, q.h.s. or q.H.S. mistaken for every hour. All can result in a dosing error	Write out "half-strength" or "at bedtime"
t.i.w. or T.I.W. (for three times a week)	Mistaken for three times a day or twice weekly resulting in an overdose	Write "3 times weekly" or "three times weekly"
s.c. or S.C. s.q. or S.Q. (for subcutaneous)	Mistaken as SL for sublingual, or "5 every" and the Q mistaken for "every"	Write "subcutaneous" or "subcutaneously"
D/C (for discharge)	Interpreted as discontinue whatever medications follow (typically discharge meds)	Write "discharge"
cc (for cubic centimeter)	Mistaken for U (units) when poorly written	Write "mL" for milliliters
A.S., A.D., A.U. (Latin abbreviation for left, right, or both ears)	Mistaken for OS, OD, and OU, etc.)	Write "left ear," "right ear," or "both ears"

ISMP "Dangerous Abbreviations" List

As indicated earlier in this chapter, the original list of dangerous abbreviations was generated by the ISMP, a nonprofit organization of pharmacists, nurses, and physicians who work collaboratively with government agencies to promote safe medication practices. Although the Joint Commission has pulled from this list its standards for NPSG 2, as outlined previously, it still strongly recommends the adoption of policies related to all the abbreviations on the ISMP list below. AAMT recommends that transcriptionists adopt the corrections recommended for the full ISMP list (provided in Appendix B of the BOS) even if ultimately their facilities and/or employers require adoption of only the minimum list indicated by the Joint Commission. In other words, it is better to err on the side of caution by knowing and applying all corrections for dangerous abbreviations. Thus, in addition to the JCAHO list of abbreviations provided in the previous section, the remaining entries recommended by ISMP are provided below.

Abbreviation/Dose Expression	Intended Meaning	Misinterpretation	Correction
Apothecary symbols	dram minim	Misunderstood or misread (symbol for dram misread for "3" and minim misread as "mL")	Use the metric system
ARA A	vidarabine	cytarabine (ARA C)	Use the complete spelling for all drug names
AZT	zidovudine (Retrovir)	azathioprine	
CPZ	Compazine (prochlorperazine)	chlorpromazine	
DPT	Demerol-Phenergan-Thorazine	diphtheria-pertussis-tetanus (vaccine)	
HCl	hydrochloric acid	potassium chloride (The "H" is mis-interpreted as "K.")	
HCT	hydrocortisone	hydrochlorothiazide	
HCTZ	hydrochlorothiazide	hydrocortisone (seen as HCT250 mg)	
MTX	methotrexate	mitoxantrone	
TAC	triamcinolone	tetracaine, Adrenalin, cocaine	
$ZnSO_4$	zinc sulfate	morphine sulfate	
"Nitro" drip	nitroglycerin infusion	sodium nitroprusside infusion	
"Norflox"	norfloxacin	Norflex	
per os	orally	The "os" can be mistaken for "left eye"	Use "p.o.," "by mouth," or "orally"
qn	nightly or at bedtime	Misinterpreted as "qh" (every hour)	Use "nightly"
qhs	nightly at bedtime	Misread as every hour	Use "nightly"

q6PM, etc.	every evening at 6 p.m.	Misread as every six hours	Use 6 p.m "nightly"
U or u	unit	Read as a zero (0) or a four (4), causing a 10-fold overdose or greater (4U seen as "40" or 4u seen as 44")	"Unit" has no acceptable abbreviation; use "unit"
x3d	for three days	Mistaken for "three doses"	Use "for three days"
BT	bedtime	Mistaken as "BID" (twice daily)	Use "at bedtime"
ss	sliding scale (insulin) or ½ (apothecary)	Mistaken for "55"	Spell out "sliding scale;" use "one-half" or use "½"
> and <	greater than and less than	Mistakenly used opposite of intended	Use "greater than" or "less than"
/ (slash mark)	separates two doses or indicates "per"	Misunderstood as the number 1 ("25 unit/10 units" read as "110" units)	Do not use a slash mark to separate doses; use "per"
Name letters and dose numbers run together (e.g., Inderal40 mg)	Inderal 40 mg	Misread as Inderal 140 mg	Always use space between drug name, dose, and unit of measure

The Final Word

To a new transcription student, these lists of dangerous abbreviations may make little sense without the dictation in which you will ultimately encounter them. As with many other concepts to which you will be introduced in both the BOS and this accompanying text, the only way to successfully learn these abbreviations is the old-fashioned way: memorize them. It may help to create flashcards for that purpose and get together with other students to quiz each other.

Regardless of the method for absorbing them, it is critical to do so. Although some standards you will learn in this text do not have a significant impact on patient outcomes, *this one does.* These abbreviations have been deemed dangerous by authorities who evaluate risk management and patient safety, and every member of the healthcare team, from provider to transcriptionist, needs to be aware of them. As mentioned previously, many providers will continue to dictate the dangerous forms out of habit, and the responsibility for recognizing and editing them appropriately will fall on the shoulders of the MT.

QUICK REVIEW

DANGEROUS ABBREVIATION	CHANGE TO:
1. Apothecary symbols	The metric system
2. > and <	"greater than" or "less than"
3. AD, A.D.	"right ear"
4. AS, A.S.	"left ear"
5. AU, A.U.	"both ears"
6. BT, b.t.	"bedtime"
7. cc, c.c.	"mL"
8. D/C	"discontinue" or "discharge"
9. Drug name abbreviations	Complete spelling
10. h.s., H.S., q.h.s.	"nightly" or "at bedtime" or "half strength"
11. µg (microgram)	"mcg"
12. o.d., O.D. (once daily)	"daily"
13. per os	"p.o." or "by mouth" or "orally"
14. q.d., Q.D.	"daily" or "every day"
15. q.6p.m., q6PM	"6 p.m. nightly"
16. q.n., qn	"nightly" or "at bedtime"
17. q.o.d., Q.O.D.	"every other day"
18. sc, SC, sq, SQ	"subcutaneous"
19. / (slash)	"per" (to separate doses)
20. ss	"sliding scale"
21. t.i.w., T.I.W.	"3 times a week"
22. U, u	"unit" or "units"
23. IU	"unit" or "units"
24. x3d	"times 3 days" or "for 3 days"
25. Zero after decimal (1.0)	Drop decimal and zero
26. Zero before decimal (.5 mg)	Always add, even if not dictated

Test Your Knowledge

Correct the following excerpts in the space provided.

1. The child is to be given Cortisporin-TC 3 mg AU twice a day.

2. The patient was changed from per-os feedings to tube feedings.

3. He was given MgSO4 intravenously upon admission.

4. ESTIMATED BLOOD LOSS: 200 cc.

5. Prior to discharge, she was started on Lanophyllin elixir 80 mg/15 mL.

6.   I am recommending Lantus SQ insulin 100 IU/mL.

_____

_____

_____

7.   MEDICATIONS: Xanax .5 mg q.h.s.

_____

_____

_____

8.   The wound measured 3.0 cm in length.

_____

_____

_____

9.   The patient responded well to intravenous nitro by IV drip.

_____

_____

_____

10.   At the time of D/C, the patient was doing well and ready to go home.

_____

_____

_____

Test Your Knowledge

Answers

1. The child is to be given Cortisporin-TC 3 mg **in both ears twice a day.**

2. The patient was changed from **oral** feedings to tube feedings.

3. He was given **magnesium sulfate** intravenously upon admission.

4. ESTIMATED BLOOD LOSS: 200 **mL.**

5. Prior to discharge, she was started on Lanophyllin elixir 80 mg **per** 15 mL.

6. I am recommending Lantus **subcutaneous** insulin 100 **units/**mL.

7. MEDICATIONS: Xanax **0.5** mg **at bedtime.**

8. The wound measured **3** cm in length.

9. The patient responded well to intravenous **nitroglycerin** by IV drip.

10. At the time of **discharge,** the patient was doing well and ready to go home.

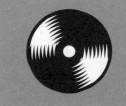

APPLICATION TEST
Take the application test for this chapter on your CD-ROM.
Access the section for
Chapter 2: "Dangerous Abbreviations."

Acceptable Forms, Back Formations, and Slang

One of the inevitable questions that arises when addressing the rules and exceptions for abbreviations: how will I know if an abbreviation or brief form is acceptable? Certainly, it can be difficult to get a handle on the rules for expanding or retaining, capitalizing, and punctuating these abbreviated terms if you are unfamiliar with the terms themselves and their general use and adoption in the healthcare setting.

As will be true of many concepts in this text, it is important to understand that medical language, like all languages, is a breathing, evolving entity. The point at which an abbreviation, term, or phrase becomes "acceptable" is difficult to pinpoint, and references and resources will not always agree on the status of that new abbreviation, term, or phrase. Fundamentally, it is usage that determines the adoption and evolution of newly coined terms and/or abbreviations derived from those terms. This can be frustrating to anyone trying to master the language, because a slang term or unacceptable abbreviation at a given point in time will likely evolve through usage to an acceptable status and then finally to formal inclusion in lexicographic texts. A new medical term is quite like a piece of legislation. It starts out as one person's idea and then generates momentum through reference by others until it either evolves to formal adoption or fizzles out and is forgotten.

Going Deeper

In the healthcare setting, a transcriptionist will begin to recognize over time whether a term or abbreviation he or she is hearing in dictation is one commonly used by others or is an obvious shortcut or faulty word construction on the part of that particular dictator. Many providers, in an effort to document quickly, will coin new terms, insert back formations, or abbreviate sections of the report that are not typically abbreviated. Again, the ultimate goal in evaluating these scenarios is to promote clarity, and experience and good judgment will assist you in making the right decisions when those situations arise.

This chapter is designed to provide a framework for differentiating acceptable abbreviations and brief forms from the faulty back formations and slang that will require editing. The information provided is by no means exhaustive, and you should always consult appropriate references when in doubt. Many abbreviation books, such as *Stedman's Abbreviations, Acronyms & Symbols*, will identify slang terms in a separate color to assist the reader in determining acceptability.

Rules & Exceptions

Acceptable Forms and Symbols

The following sections deal with specific abbreviations, brief forms, and symbols encountered in healthcare documentation that are commonly used and are generally acceptable to transcribe in abbreviated form except in sections of the report where all abbreviations must be expanded (see Chapter 1) and where otherwise specified for reasons related to clarity.

a.k.a.   Abbreviation meaning *also known as*. Use lowercase letters with periods to distinguish from *AKA*, meaning *above-knee amputation*.

> **The report was published by the National Academies, a.k.a. National Academy of Sciences, National Academy of Engineering, National Research Council, Institute of Medicine.**

a.m, AM, p.m., PM

Acceptable abbreviations for ante meridiem (before noon) and post meridiem (after noon), with the lowercase forms being preferred. Formal publications use small capitals, which, if available, may also be used in transcription.

> **8:15 a.m.** *or* **8:15 AM**

Do not use these abbreviations with a phrase such as *in the morning, in the evening, tonight, o'clock.*

> **8:15 a.m.** *not* **8:15 a.m. o'clock**
> **10:30 PM** *not* **10:30 PM in the evening**

Use periods with *a.m.* and *p.m.* so that *a.m.* won't be misread as the word *am.* Do not use periods with the uppercase *AM* and *PM.* Insert a space between the numerals preceding these abbreviations and the abbreviations themselves, but do not use spaces within the abbreviations.

> **11 a.m.** *or* **11 AM**
> *not* **11a.m.** *or* **11AM**
> *not* **11 a. m.** *or* **11 A M**

ampersand (&) Symbol meaning *and.* Use with certain single-letter abbreviations separated by *and.* Do not space before or after the ampersand. Do not use ampersand forms in operative titles or diagnoses. Check appropriate references to identify other acceptable uses.

> **D&C**
> **T&A**

BPM, bpm Abbreviation for *beats per minute*.

> Pulse: 70 beats per minute.
>
> *or* Pulse: 70 BPM.
>
> *or* Pulse: 70 bpm.

BP Abbreviation for *blood pressure*.

> DICTATED
> **Blood pressure 110/80.**
>
> TRANSCRIBED
> **Blood pressure 110/80.**
> *or* **BP 110/80.**

blood types Write out *B negative* and *B positive* rather than *B−* or *B+* because the minus or plus sign is easily overlooked.

degrees (°) In expressing angles in orthopedics, write out *degrees* or use the degree sign (°).

> The patient was able to straight leg raise to 40 degrees.
>
> *or* The patient was able to straight leg raise to 40°.

Use the degree sign (°) in imaging studies and temperature expressions.

> Positioning the patient's head at a 90° angle allowed for efficient acquisition of data over a 180° arc.
>
> Temperature was 99.1°F.

If the symbol is not available, spell out *degree* or *degrees*.

ditto marks
Do not use ditto marks (") to indicate *the same*; instead, repeat the term or phrase. Do not use ditto marks as a symbol for *inches*, except in tables as a space-saving device.

> **The infant was 22 inches long.**
>
> *not* **The infant was 22" long.**

division symbol
Do not use the division symbol (÷) except in tables and mathematical expressions.

DNR
A DNR (do not resuscitate) order is placed in a patient's chart when either the patient or the family has indicated that no emergency resuscitative measures are to be employed.

> **His status was changed to DNR yesterday.**

Dr., Dr
Courtesy title for doctors. Use only for earned doctorates (medical or other), not honorary doctorates. The use of an ending period is optional.

> **Dr. Brown**
> **Dr. C. Everett Koop**
>
> *not* **Dr. George W. Bush**

Use *Dr.* not *Doctor* in salutations unless the salutation is directed to more than one doctor. Do not use *Drs.* as a plural form in salutations; write out *Doctors* instead.

> **Dear Dr. Watson:**
> **Dear Doctors Watson and Crick:**

Do not use *Dr.* or *Doctor* when credentials are given.

> **John Brown, MD**
>
> *not* **Dr. John Brown, MD**

drug terminology

Use lowercase abbreviations with periods for Latin abbreviations that are related to doses and dosages. Do not use abbreviations found on the "Dangerous Abbreviations" list from ISMP (see Chapter 2). Avoid using all capitals because they emphasize the abbreviation rather than the drug name. Avoid lowercase abbreviations without periods because some may be misread as words. Do not translate.

Abbreviation	Latin Phrase	English Translation
a.c.	Ante cibum	Before food
b.i.d.	Bis in die	Twice a day
gtt.	Guttae	Drops (spell out)
n.p.o.	Nil per os	Nothing by mouth
n.r.	Non repetatur	Do not repeat
p.c.	Post cibum	After food
p.o.	Per os	By mouth
p.r.n.	Pro re nata	As needed
q.4 h.	Quaque 4 hora	Every 4 hours
q.h.	Quaque hora	Every hour
q.i.d.	Quarter in die	Four times a day
t.i.d.	Ter in die	Three times a day
u.d.	Ut dictum	As directed

Where?
BOS pp. 146–147

BOS Statement

Note: We have inserted a space after the numeral *4* in *q.4 h.* on the advice of ISMP so that the number is more easily and clearly read. Invalid Latin abbreviations such as *q.a.m. (every morning)* and mixed Latin and English abbreviations such as *q.4 hours (every 4 hours)* have become commonplace. However, as with all abbreviations, avoid those that are obscure (like *a.c.b. for before breakfast)* or dangerous. For example, *b.i.w.* is both obscure **and** dangerous. It is intended to mean *twice weekly* but it could be mistaken for *twice daily*, resulting in a dosage frequency seven times that intended.

Note: AAMT continues to discourage the dropping of periods in lowercase abbreviations that might be misread as words (for example, *bid* and *tid*). If you must drop the periods, use all capitals, but keep in mind that the overuse of capitals, particularly in relation to drug doses and dosages, would draw more attention to the capitalized abbreviations than to the drug names themselves.

equal, equal to Do not use the equal symbol (=) except in tables and mathematical presentations.

exam Acceptable brief form for *examination* when dictated, except as a heading.

> **The physical exam was negative.**
>
> **PHYSICAL EXAMINATION**
> **HEENT: Head normal.**
> **NECK: Supple.**

geographic names State and territory names may be abbreviated when they are preceded by a city name, and country names may be abbreviated when preceded by a city, state, or territory name.

> **Orlando, FL**
> **Washington, DC**

Do not abbreviate names of states, territories, countries or similar units within reports when they stand alone. However, abbreviations **may** be used in addresses, and **should** be used when addressing an envelope.

> **The patient moved here 3 years ago from Canada.**

greater, less than, greater than The word *greater* is overused in medical parlance and is often dictated inappropriately when *more*, *longer*, or *over* would be a better choice of words. As so often happens, shorthand is used in a handwritten patient chart, and a dictating physician will read the chart while dictating and will use the words that go with the shorthand symbol, when that may not be the best translation of the symbol.

> DICTATED
> **The pain persisted greater than 24 hours.**
>
> TRANSCRIBED
> **The pain persisted longer than 24 hours.**

The greater than (>) and less than (<) symbols are often mistaken for their opposite sign in meaning, and ISMP advises against their use.

> **The patient's performance on the trial is in the impaired range (289 seconds, less than the 1st percentile).**
>
> **She weighed less than 100 pounds.**
>
> **The patient exhibited greater lung capacity following treatments.**

Greek letters Spell out the English translation when the word stands alone. Do not capitalize English translations. Use the Greek letter or spell it out when it is part of an extended term, according to the preferred form; consult appropriate references for guidance.

> **alpha** α
> **beta** β
> **gamma** γ

In extended terms, use of a hyphen after the Greek letter is optional, but the hyphen is not used after the English translation.

> **β-globulin *or* B globulin**
> **beta globulin**

International System of Units

Where?
BOS pp. 214–215

BOS Statement

The International System of Units (SI) is the system of metric measurements adopted in 1960 at the Eleventh General Conference on Weights and Measures of the International Organization for Standards. Since the 1977 recommendation of the 30th World Health Assembly that SI units be used in medicine, some medical journals use the SI to a limited degree, some use it only in conjunction with conventional units, and some have not yet adopted it.

The adoption of SI in documentation of patient care is likewise sporadic, but it is sufficiently widespread, in whole or part, to warrant the attention of medical transcriptionists. It should be noted that, although some units from the apothecary system remain in use, all elements of the apothecary system have been dropped from the compendium of the United States Pharmacopeia (USP) system.

Additionally, the accelerated movement toward international adoption of the electronic patient record is likely to strengthen the adoption of the SI in order to facilitate communication across borders.

Basic Units and Properties of the SI

Base Unit	SI symbol	Basic Property
meter	m	length
kilogram	kg	mass
second	s	time
ampere	A	electric current
kelvin	K	thermodynamic temperature

candela	cd	luminous intensity
mole	mol	amount of substance
radian	rad	plane angle
steradian	sr	solid angle

Basic Units Derived From SI Basic Units

Derived Unit	Name and Symbol
area	square meter (m^2)
volume	cubic meter (m^3)
frequency	hertz (Hz)
work, energy	joule (J)
pressure	pascal (Pa)
force	newton (N)
density	kilogram per cubic meter (kg/m^3)
speed, velocity	meter per second (m/s)
acceleration	meter per second squared (m/s^2)
electric field strength	volt per meter (V/m)

Abbreviate most units of measure that accompany numerals and include virgule (/) constructions. Use the same abbreviation for singular and plural forms. Do not use periods with abbreviated units of measure.

1 g
20 g
40 mm/h

Do not abbreviate English units of time except in virgule (/) constructions. Do not use periods with such abbreviations.

minute	min
week	wk
month	mo

> **hour**   **h**
> **day**   **d**
> **year**   **y**
> **The patient is 5 days old.**
> **He will return in 1 week for followup.**
> **40 mm/h**

Jr., Jr; Sr., Sr   Abbreviations for *junior* and *senior* in names. Usage of a comma before and a period after is optional, but use both or neither. Do not use all capitals (JR, SR).

> **Dr. Martin Luther King, Jr.**
>
> *or* **Dr. Martin Luther King Jr**

Latin abbreviations   These Latin abbreviations are commonly used in English communications and need not be translated, although the medical transcriptionist should understand their meaning before using them.

Abbreviation	Latin	English
e.g. *or* eg	exempli gratia	for example
et al. *or* et al	et alii	and others
etc. *or* etc	et cetera	and so forth
i.e. *or* ie	id est	that is
viz. *or* viz	videlicet	that is, namely

MD   Abbreviation for *Doctor of Medicine*. Preferred style is without periods. If periods are used, do not space within the abbreviation (M.D., not M. D.).

mEq   Abbreviation for *milliequivalent*. Use with numerals. Do not use periods. Do not add *s* for plural.

> **20 mEq**

mg%   Abbreviation for *milligrams percent*. Equivalent to milligrams per deciliter (mg/dL), which is the preferred nomenclature, but transcribe as dictated. Do not use periods. Do not space between *mg* and %.

minus, minus sign (–) Write out the word *minus* if you are not certain the symbol will be noticeable or clear. Write out *minus* to indicate below-zero temperatures.

> **minus 40, −40**
>
> ***but* minus 38 degrees**
>
> ***not* −38 degrees**

mmHg Abbreviation for *millimeters of mercury*. Use with pressure readings (blood pressure, tourniquet pressure, etc.). Need not use if not dictated.

negative sign (–) Do not use except in tables or special applications, e.g., blood nomenclature. Also avoid if its usage may cause the reader to overlook it.

> **blood type O negative**
>
> ***preferred to* blood type O–**

percent (%) Note that *percent* is a singe word. Do not use the abbreviation *pct.* except in tables. Instead, use % or *percent*. Use the symbol % after a numeral. Do not space between the numeral and the symbol.

> **13% monos, 1% bands**
>
> **She has had a 10% increase in weight since her last visit.**
>
> **MCHC 34%**
>
> **10% solution**

Use numerals for the number preceding %. When the number is written out, as at the beginning of a sentence, write out *percent*.

> 50%
>
> *not* fifty %

plus, plus sign (+)

Do not use the plus sign without a numeral.

> +1, +2, +3
> *or* 1+, 2+, 3+
> *not* +, ++, +++

In laboratory or technical readings, use the symbol unless it will not be noticeable or clear.

> **3+ gram-positive cocci**

subcu

Abbreviated form for *subcutaneous* or *subcuticular*. When "subcu" is dictated and you are unsure which term is intended, spell *subcu* or *subcut*. Do not use the abbreviation *sub q* because the *q* can be mistaken for a medication dosage [see Chapter 2].

> DICTATED & TRANSCRIBED
>
> **The wound was closed with running subcu stitches of 5-0 Prolene.**

units of measure

Metric system: system of weights and measures based upon the meter.

deci-	one-tenth
centi-	one-hundredth
milli-	one-thousandth
micro-	one-millionth
nano-	one-billionth
pico-	one-trillionth
deka-	10 units
hecto-	100 units
kilo-	1000 units
mega-	one million units

| giga- | one billion units |
| tera- | one trillion units |

Abbreviations for metric units commonly used in medical reports:

cm	centimeter
dL	deciliter
g	gram
L	liter
mEq	milliequivalents
mg	milligram
mL	milliliter
mm	millimeter
mmHg	millimeter of mercury
mmol	millimole
msec, ms	millisecond

Nonmetric units: spell out nonmetric units of measure (*ounce, pound, inch, foot, yard, mile,* etc.) to express weight, depth, distance, height, length, and width, except in tables.

4 pounds
5 ounces
14 inches
5 feet
5 feet 3 inches, *not* **5'3"** *or* **5 ft. 3 in.**

X, x

Use only with numerals. Use a lowercase *x* in expressions of area and volume, as a multiplication symbol, and when it takes the place of the word *times*. A capital X is generally used to express magnification. Use a lowercase *x* to express *by* in dimensions. When the word "times" is dictated and can be translated as *for*, it should be transcribed as *for* rather than *times* or *x*. When the word "times" is dictated and means the number of times a thing was done, the letter *x* can be used.

X30 magnification
13 x 2 cm

DICTATED
The patient was given antibiotics to take times 2 weeks.

TRANSCRIBED
The patient was given antibiotics to take *for* 2 weeks.

Blood cultures were negative x3.

Language to Avoid

BOS Statement

Where?
BOS pp. 234–237

Modern medicine is constantly evolving and so is its language. In addition, with the fast pace of American health care, clinicians sometimes find themselves dictating their notes on the fly, before they have had a chance to put their thoughts together. The result may be an awkward use of language and frequent neologisms (newly formed words).

Sometimes a noun or adjective is used as a verb. If possible, edit awkwardly created verbs.

DICTATED
Stool was guaiac'd.

TRANSCRIBED
Stool guaiac test was done.

Likewise, if possible, edit proper nouns dictated as verbs.

DICTATED
The baby was de-lee'd on the abdomen.

TRANSCRIBED
The baby was suctioned on the abdomen using a DeLee.

back formation

New word formed by altering an existing word (usually a noun). Back formations are often verbs but may appear as adjectives or adverbs. They are frequently encountered in medical dictation. Use dictated back formations if they have become acceptable through widespread use. Avoid absurd back formations or ones that will be confusing to the reader. It is difficult to say which back formations will never become accepted; this is ultimately determined by usage. False verbs and other back formations are increasingly prevalent in the communications industry and technical world, but they should be used judiciously in transcribed health records.

Original Word	Back Formation
dehiscence	to dehisce
diagnosis	to diagnose
torsion	to torse

coined terms

Non-official, non-standard terms. Many are back formations. Avoid as much as possible and consult resources when you are uncertain.

We *lased* the tattoo in one session. *(removed by laser)*

jargon

Special language that is used and fully understood only by members of a particular craft, trade, or profession. Like other jargons, that of the healthcare professions parallels, but only slightly overlaps, formal technical terminology. It consists partly of lay and technical terms to which special meanings are assigned. It is largely unrecorded in reference books and is highly informal, including some expressions that are slangy and humorous. Medical jargon tends to be particularly imprecise and may be offensive and derogatory.

DICTATED
urines

TRANSCRIBED
urine samples

language to rewrite

Leave blank and flag obscenities, derogatory or inflammatory remarks, and double entendres (words or word combinations, symbols and abbreviations that have varying, and usually inappropriate, meanings).

> DICTATED
> **He is complaining of some SOB.**
>
> TRANSCRIBED
> **He is complaining of some shortness of breath.**

Test Your Knowledge

Indicate the abbreviation for the following words and phrases in the blank provided.

1.   millimeters of mercury

2.   twice a day

3.   milliliters

4.   after food

5.   also known as

6.   as needed

7.   hertz

8.   moles

9.   subcutaneous

10.   for example

Each of the following sentences contains one or more incorrectly transcribed abbreviation, symbol, or brief form. Correct the sentences in the space provided.

11. HEIGHT: 5' 6 " and weight 140 lbs.

12. She was given 20 milliequivalents of potassium by injection.

13. The patient was referred by Dr. Edward Smith, MD, for consultation.

14. The temperature today is −15 degrees.

15. The patient reportedly took >100 Tylenol.

Test Your Knowledge

Answers

1.	mmHg
2.	b.i.d.
3.	mL
4.	p.c.
5.	a.k.a.
6.	p.r.n.
7.	Hz
8.	mol
9.	subcu *or* subcut
10.	e.g.
11.	HEIGHT: 5 feet 6 inches and 140 pounds.
12.	She was given 20 mEq of potassium by injection.
13.	The patient was referred by Dr. Edward Smith for consultation. *or* The patient was referred by Edward Smith, MD, for consultation.
14.	The temperature today is minus 15 degrees. *or* The temperature today is minus 15°.
15.	The patient reportedly took more than 100 Tylenol.

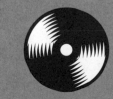

APPLICATION TEST
Take the application test for this chapter on your CD-ROM.
Access the section for
Chapter 3: "Acceptable Forms, Back Formations, and Slang."

Quantifiers

Cardinal and Ordinal Numbers
Rules and Exceptions

BOS Statement

Numerals, or figures, stand out from the surrounding text and serve a functional purpose in medical reports, where they should be used almost exclusively as opposed to spelled-out numbers.

Where?
BOS p. 276

> **She was seen in the emergency room 1 hour after the accident.**
>
> **He tried 3 different medications without success.**
>
> **The specimen weighed less than 2 pounds.**

Exceptions: There are always exceptions to any rule, and judgment and discretion are needed when deciding whether to use numerals or spell out numbers.

Going Deeper

At the heart of patient encounter documentation is the quantifying information that enables the healthcare team to diagnose, treat, and manage patients. There is arguably no more critical information recorded and relied upon than the numeric values that represent a wide variety of indicators for both cause and effect in managing disease. Whether it is the patient's age, vital signs, duration of symptoms, wound measurements, laboratory values, drug dosages, length of stay, indication of pain, or classification of disease, numbers are a critical part of the patient record. They need to be communicated clearly and accurately in all areas of the report, and they represent an area of tremendous potential error in the record.

The rules and exceptions outlined in this chapter for cardinal and ordinal numbers should be learned and applied well. Like the dangerous abbreviations indicated in Chapter 2, the erroneous transcription of a number can lead to potential risk management and continuity of care issues that must be carefully addressed.

As in other areas of style and standards, when determining how a particular dictated value should be transcribed, clarity of expression will always be the single driving factor.

It will be important to understand in approaching this material that the rules for numbers you learned as a child in school will likely not apply in this setting. Many were taught to spell out all numbers under the number 10 and to use the numeric (arabic) value for all numbers greater than 9. However, in the clinical setting, numbers need to be read and communicated quickly and clearly. Spelling out numeric values, even under the number 10, is not considered the most efficient way to communicate them to the many care providers who may ultimately read and/or scan the document. Remember, while the patient record is a formal, legal document, its primary function in the healthcare setting is to communicate information that contributes to the ongoing treatment and care of the patient. In formal writing (for publication, for example), it is still the preference to spell out numbers under 10, but your traditional understanding of formality needs to be weighed against the greater need for clarity where medical transcription is concerned. Therefore, since numeric values that stand out on the page are less likely to be overlooked or misinterpreted, the standard is to use them in transcription.

There are exceptions, of course, where numbers are dictated at the beginning of the sentence or adjacent to other numeric values. The rules for managing those exceptions are provided below, and you will need to let these rules, and an understanding of clarity, guide you through those exceptions.

Facility Policy   As with other points of style and standards, provider/client preference will often be the final word on this issue, though it is not likely that an employer or client will ask that you spell out numerals in vital areas of the report. You may, however, encounter providers who are well published or are particularly formal in the letters they dictate. They might require you to use the old rule of spelling out numbers under 10 in their correspondence, but again, any numeric values (such as vital signs, laboratory values, or drug dosages) should still be expressed with numerals, even in correspondence.

Values   While they are not covered in this text, it is important to note that knowing and understanding normal value ranges for common laboratory tests, doses for commonly prescribed medications, and the numeric ranges of common surgical instruments and materials can assist you in knowing how to apply the rules for numbers encountered in this chapter and the rest of this unit. For example, knowing that Lanoxin, a cardiac glycoside antiarrhythmic, is commonly dosed at 0.125 and 0.25 mg will predispose you to transcribing the leading zero and decimal even if it is unclearly dictated or if it is rapidly dictated as "Lanoxin 1-2-5," as is sometimes the case. Likewise, when you hear a physician dictate, "Specific gravity ten twenty," your deeper understanding of urinalysis laboratory values and the normal range for specific gravity (1.005 to 1.030) will lead you to correctly transcribe that value as *Specific gravity 1.020.*

In other words, memorizing these rules alone will not always enable you to correctly transcribe a numeric value. You will need to apply both these rules and knowledge of medical context to correctly represent that value in the document.

Rules & Exceptions

BOS Statement

Where?
BOS pp. 279–281

RULES

arabic v roman numerals

There is a trend away from the use of roman numerals and toward the use of arabic numerals. A good example of this is in diabetes terminology, where an international expert committee dropped the roman numerals in favor of arabic, noting the danger of a roman numeral *II* being misread as an arabic number *11*. In addition, the *AMA Manual of Style* states, "Avoid the use of roman numerals except when part of established nomenclature."

arabic numerals

The arabic numerals are 0, 1, 2, 3, 4, 5, 6, 7, 8, 9.

Most numerals used in medicine are expressed as arabic numerals. Therefore, a general rule is to use arabic numerals unless roman numerals are specified or unless there is strong documentation that the preferred form is roman.

Grades are generally written in arabic numerals.

> **grade 3/6 holosystolic murmur**
> **CIN grade 3**
> **grade 3 chondromalacia patellae**

See roman numerals *below, as well as* cancer classifications (Chapter 15), classification systems (Chapter 9), *and* orthopedics (Chapter 17).

roman numerals

Do not use periods with roman numerals. Seven letters make up the roman numeral system. Capital letters are used except in special circumstances; e.g., lowercase letters (i, v, x, etc.) are used as page numbers for preliminary material (contents pages, preface, etc.) in a book.

```
I   = 1
V   = 5
X   = 10
L   = 50
C   = 100
D   = 500
M   = 1000
```

When a letter follows a letter of greater value, it increases the value of the preceding letter.

VI   (5 + 1 = 6)

When a letter precedes a letter of greater value it diminishes the value of the following letter.

IV   (5 - 1 = 4)

A bar over a letter indicates multiplication by 1000.

$\overline{X}$ = 10,000

(Following are some common applications that use roman numerals. To determine arabic or roman numeral usage for other applications, check the arabic section of this topic and several other entries throughout this book, as well as other appropriate references [especially word books in the medical specialty involved].)

Stages are generally expressed with roman numerals, although there are exceptions.

stage IV decubitus ulcer
ovarian carcinoma, FIGO stage II
stage 3 Garden fracture of femoral neck

HINT: Many instructors help students remember the rule for roman numerals with stages by encouraging them to think of "Romans on a stage."

Classifications. Some classifications that are not expressed in stages also use roman numerals. Examples: NYHA classification of heart failure, Clark levels for malignant melanoma

> **Clark level II**
> **Cardiac failure, class III**

EKG standard bipolar leads. The three bipolar leads on a standard (12-lead) EKG are transcribed with roman numerals.

> **lead I, lead II, lead III**

Cranial nerves. Arabic or roman numerals may be used.

> **cranial nerves 1-12 *or* cranial nerves I-XII**

Wars, people, animals. Roman numerals are generally used for wars, people, and animals.

> **World War II**
> **Henry Ford III**
> **Rover II**
> ***but* C. Roy Post 4th *(the personal preference of this cereal magnate)***

ordinals

Ordinal numbers are used to indicate order or position in a series rather than quantity.

Ordinals are commonly spelled out, especially when the series goes no higher than 10 items. However, as with all numbers in medical reports, AAMT recommends using numerals: 1st, 2nd, 3rd, 4th, etc.

Do not use a period with ordinal numbers.

> 3rd rib (*or* third)
> 5th finger (*or* fifth)
> She is to return for her 3rd (*or* third) visit in
> 2 days.
> She was in her 9th (*or* ninth) month of pregnancy.
> His return visits are scheduled for the 15th and
> 25th of next month.
> The 4th cranial nerve...

punctuation

Hyphens. Use hyphens when numbers are used with words as compound modifiers preceding nouns.

> **2-pillow orthopnea**
> **13-year 2-month-old girl**

Use hyphens to join some compound nouns with numbers as prefixes. Check appropriate references for specific terms.

> **2-D**

Use hyphens in compound numbers from 21 to 99 when they are written out. (Note: The only time they should be written out is at the beginning of a sentence.)

> **thirty-four**
> **one hundred fifty-three**

Commas. Use a comma to separate groups of three numerals in numbers of 5 digits or more, but omit the commas if decimals are used. The comma in 4-digit numerals may be omitted.

> **Platelet count was 354,000.**
> **White count was 7100.** *or*
> **White count was 7,100.**
> **12345.67**

Do not place commas between words expressing a number.

> **four hundred forty-eight**
> *not* **four hundred, forty-eight**

plurals

Use 's to form the plural of single-digit numerals.

> **4 x 4's**

Add *s* without an apostrophe to form the plural of multiple-digit numbers, including years.

> **She is in her 20s.**
> **She was born in the 1940s.**

multiple digits

When dictated in a form such as "four point two thousand" or "five point eight million," numerals may be transcribed in one of two ways:

> **4.2 thousand**
> *or* **4200**
>
> **5.8 million**
> *or* **5,800,000**

proper names

Use words or figures for numbers in proper names, according to the entity's preference.

> **20th Century Insurance**
> **Three Dollar Cafe**

at end of line

When possible, do not separate numerals from the terms they accompany. Do not allow a numeral to end on one line and its accompanying term to begin the next.

> ....grade 2.
> *not*
> ....grade
> 2.

It is important to note that using a hard return to facilitate this could interfere with the upload of the document on many field-driven documentation platforms, so AAMT recommends using a nonbreaking space between the term and its accompanying value. In an MS Word environment, for example, this is facilitated by using the Ctrl, Shift, and space bar keys simultaneously.

EXCEPTIONS

adjacent numbers

When two numbers are consecutive, spell out one of them to avoid confusion.

> **The patient was instructed to drink four 8-ounce glasses of water a day.**
>
> **Discharge Medication: Os-Cal 500 one daily.**
>
> **two 8-inch drains**

Use a comma to separate adjacent unrelated numerals if neither can be readily expressed in words and the sentence cannot be readily reworded.

> **In March 2002, 2038 patients were seen in the emergency room.**

fractions

Spell out or use numerals for common fractions. Use the dictation style as a guide.

> **An hour and a half before presentation, the patient slipped and fell.**
>
> *or* **Approximately 1-1/2 hours before presentation...** *(if dictated "one and a half hours" or "one and one-half hours")*

> The glass was two-thirds full. *or* The glass was 2/3 full.
>
> 7/8-inch wound
>
> a half-inch incision *or* a 1/2-inch incision *(since it was dictated precisely)*
>
> about a half inch below the sternal notch *(the word* about *makes this an imprecise measurement)*
>
> He smokes a pack and a half of cigarettes per day. *or* He smokes 1½ packs of cigarettes per day. *or* He smokes 1-1/2 packs of cigarettes per day.

beginning of a sentence

Spell out numbers that begin a sentence, or recast the sentence.

> DICTATED
> **Fourteen days ago she started having severe cramping.**
>
> TRANSCRIBED
> **Fourteen days ago she started having severe cramping.** *or* **She started having severe cramping 14 days ago.**

An exception to this exception: A complete year that begins a sentence need not be spelled out.

> **2005 will mark our hospital's 100th anniversary.**

NOTE: Although it's acceptable to begin a sentence with a year, it is better to recast the sentence if possible.

> DICTATED
> **1995 was when her symptoms began.**
>
> TRANSCRIBED
> **Her symptoms began in 1995.**

zero

Zero is always spelled out when it stands alone.

> **The patient had zero response to the treatment.**
>
> **Her symptoms usually appear when the outside temperature drops below zero.**
>
> *but*
>
> **gravida 1, para 0**
>
> **0°F**

pronouns

Spell out numbers used as pronouns.

> **The radiologist compared the previous x-rays with the most recent one.**

numbers commonly spelled out

Common or accepted usage may dictate that a word be spelled out. For example, use of a numeral may cause confusion by placing emphasis and implying a precise quantity where none is intended.

> **His symptoms went from one extreme to the other.**
>
> **The patient was given a choice between two courses of treatment; she chose the diet and exercise over medication.**

nonspecific numbers

Spell out nonspecific (indefinite) numeric expressions.

> **She described hundreds of symptoms.** *(not 100s)*
> **Several thousand people were tested.**

HINT: The "pronoun exception" applies if you can replace the number with another word that is not a number.

The Final Word

As you acclimate to transcription and healthcare delivery, you will begin to recognize the critical components of a patient's record. You will begin to identify key inclusions and values upon which further treatment and provision of care rely. This will enable you to apply these, and other standards, consistently in your transcription. Understanding the process of healthcare delivery will be invaluable in applying all of these standards in an informed manner. Human judgment in the documentation process will always be critical to an accurate record. Often, the slightest change in a numeric value, such as the omission or misplacement of a decimal point or comma, can lead to the misinterpretation of core patient data and potentially to the misapplication of that data in a treatment context. While ultimately the provider needs to authenticate that dictation and verify its accuracy, the reality is that in an overburdened healthcare delivery system, providers are not always as careful as they should be, and they rely very heavily on medical transcriptionists to be watchful and vigilant in documenting patient care. Therefore, it is always sound practice to slow down and be extra careful when transcribing these key sections of a patient record, and of course, always flagging a report when that data is unclearly dictated or dictated in error.

QUICK REVIEW

1. Use numerals for all numeric values indicated in a patient record except:

   a. Numbers at the beginning of a sentence (*recast preferred*).

   b. Two adjacent consecutive numbers.

   c. Nonspecific references to numbers or fractional amounts.

   d. References to the number zero when it stands alone.

2. Use roman numerals for:

   a. Stages.

   b. Cranial nerves.

   c. Some classification systems (Clark levels for melanoma invasion and NYHA classes for cardiac failure).

   d. EKG bipolar leads.

   e. Wars, people, and animals

3. Use arabic numerals for all other numeric references.

4. Use numerals to express ordinal numbers.

5. Use hyphens with numbers when part of a compound modifier, when joined with a letter or word as a compound noun, and in compound numbers when they are written out.

6. Use commas to separate groups of numerals in numbers of 5 digits or more.

7. Use *'s* to pluralize single-digit numerals and *s* without the apostrophe to pluralize multiple-digit numerals.

8. Defer to entity preference when spelling out numbers or using numerals in proper names.

9. Do not separate numerals from their accompanying terms or units of measure at the end of a line of text.

Test Your Knowledge

Indicate the correct transcription of the following dictated excerpts in the space provided.

1. The police department sent their K-nine unit to the scene.

2. This is the patient's eleventh visit to the emergency room this year.

3. Examination revealed a five centimeter laceration on the right arm.

4. White count was eleven thousand with a left shift.

5. She retired in her early 60's.

6. She was admitted and diagnosed with class three cardiac failure.

_____

_____

_____

7. I elicited zero response to painful stimuli from the patient.

_____

_____

_____

8. She was given four fifteen milligram Toradol to take home at discharge.

_____

_____

_____

9. Three days ago she began having pain in the lower back.

_____

_____

_____

10. The procedure lasted about an hour and a half.

_____

_____

_____

Test Your Knowledge

Answers

---

1. The police department sent their K-9 unit to the scene. *(preferred style)*

---

2. This is the patient's 11th visit to the emergency room this year.

---

3. Examination revealed a 5 cm laceration on the right arm.

---

4. White count was 11,000 with a left shift.

---

5. She retired in her early 60s.

---

6. She was admitted and diagnosed with class III cardiac failure.

---

7. I elicited zero response to painful stimuli from the patient. *(correct as is)*

---

8. She was given four 15 mg Toradol to take home at discharge.

---

9. Three days ago she began having pain in the lower back.
or
She began having pain in the lower back 3 days ago.

---

10. The procedure lasted about an hour and a half. *(correct as is)*

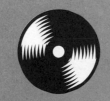

APPLICATION TEST
Take the application test for this chapter on your CD-ROM.
Access the section for
Chapter 4: "Cardinal and Ordinal Numbers."

Numeric Referents

In addition to the myriad instances in a patient report that you will encounter the numeric values covered in Chapter 4, there are other numeric referents that often occur in a dictated record, such as those related to age, money, dates, and time. The standards related to the transcription of these referents will be addressed here, and most of them will likely be familiar, as they generally do not deviate from how these referents would be represented in a nonmedical context. Given the detailed breakdown in the previous chapter as to when and where to use a numeral as opposed to spelling it out, some of these entries will seem repetitive of that information, but they address specific *Book of Style* entries that fall outside of the section on numbers and are worth repeating here.

Again, as stressed in the previous chapter, an understanding of the clinical context in which these numeric referents are encountered will empower you to recognize them and apply these standards appropriately.

Rules & Exceptions

ages
Use numerals to express ages, except at the beginning of a sentence.

> **37-year-old man**
> **3½-year-old child**
> **3-year 7-month-old girl**

at the beginning of a sentence

Recast the sentence or write out the number.

> DICTATED
> **7-year-old patient who comes in today for...**
>
> TRANSCRIBED
> **A 7-year-old patient who comes in today for...**
>
> *or* **This 7-year-old patient comes in today for...**
>
> *or* **Seven-year-old patient who comes in today for...**

as adjectival phrases

Use hyphens if the adjectival phrase precedes the noun.

> **15-year-old boy** *not* **15 year old boy**
> **13-year-olds** *not* **13 year olds**

Do not use hyphens when the phrase stands alone.

> **The patient, who is 15 years old,...**
>
> *not* **15-years-old**

Use a hyphen in a phrase in which the noun following the phrase is implied, or in a phrase that is serving as a noun. Alternatively, edit to a form that does not require hyphens.

> **The patient, a 33-year-old, was pregnant for the fifth time.**
>
> **(The word** patient *or* woman **is implied following 33-year-old.)**
>
> *or* **The patient, 33 years old, was pregnant for the fifth time.**

as decade reference

Use numerals plus *s* to refer to decades. Do not use an apostrophe.

> **The patient is in her 50s. (*not* 50's *or* fifties)**

caliber of weapons

Express with decimal point followed by arabic numerals and a hyphen. Do not place a zero before the decimal point.

> **.38-caliber pistol**

clock referents

When an anatomic position is described in terms of clockface orientation as seen by the viewer, use *o'clock* unless the position is subdivided.

> **The incision was made at the 3 o'clock position.**
>
> DICTATED
> **The cyst was found at the 2:30 o'clock position.**
>
> TRANSCRIBED
> **The cyst was found at the 2:30 position.**

dates

Punctuation. When the month, day, and year are given in this sequence, set off the year by commas. Do not use ordinals.

> **She was admitted on December 14, 2001, and discharged on January 4, 2002.**
>
> ***not* ...January 4th, 2002 *(4th is an ordinal)***

Do not use commas when the month and year are given without the day, or when the military date sequence (day, month, year) is used.

> **She was admitted in December 2001 and discharged in January 2002.**
>
> **She was admitted on 14 December 2001 and discharged on 4 January 2002.**

Do not use punctuation after the year if the date stands alone, as in admission and discharge dates on reports.

> **Admission date: April 4, 2000**
>
> **Discharge date: April 5, 2000**

Ordinals. Use ordinals when the day of the month precedes the month and is preceded by *the*; do not use commas. Do not use ordinals in month/day/year format.

> **the 4th of April 2001** *not* **April 4th, 2001**

Military style. When the military style is used, the day precedes the month. Use numerals; do not use commas. Write out or abbreviate the month (without periods) and use arabic figures for day and year.

> **4 April 2001**
> **4 Apr 2001**

In text. It is preferable to spell out dates used in the body of a report, writing out the name of the month and using four digits for the year.

> **The patient was previously seen on April 4, 2001.**

However, if dates are used repeatedly, as in a long history or hospital course, they may be expressed as numerals separated by virgules or hyphens as long as they are clearly understood.

> **Electrolytes on April 24, 2001, revealed a sodium of 135, potassium 4.3, bicarbonate 25, chlorides 102. Repeated on 4/25 and again on 4/26, electrolytes remained within normal limits.**

When only the month and day are dictated, and not the year, add the year only if you are certain what year is being referred to.

DICTATED
The patient was last seen on April 4th.

TRANSCRIBED
The patient was last seen on April 4, 2001.
(only if you're sure it's 2001)

End of line. Divide dates at the end of a line of text between the day and the year. Avoid dividing between the month and the day.

...................................**February 17,**
2001

not

...................................**February**
17, 2001

It is important to note that using a hard return to facilitate this could interfere with the upload of the document on many field-driven documentation platforms, so AAMT recommends using a nonbreaking space between the term and its accompanying value. In an MS Word environment, for example, this is facilitated by using the Ctrl, Shift, and space bar keys simultaneously.

decimals,
decimal units

Use numerals to express decimal amounts. Use the period as a decimal point or indicator.

Metric measurements. Always use the decimal form with metric units of measure, even when they are dictated as a fraction.

DICTATED
The mass was two and a half centimeters in diameter.

TRANSCRIBED
The mass was 2.5 cm in diameter.

Exception: When the originator uses a fraction that cannot be exactly translated into decimals, transcribe as dictated.

> DICTATED
> **one third centimeter**
>
> TRANSCRIBED
> **1/3 cm**

When whole numbers are dictated, do not add a decimal point and zero because doing so may cause them to be misread. It also indicates a degree of specificity that, if not dictated, was not intended by the originator. This is critical with drug doses because the addition of a decimal point and zero could lead to serious consequences if misread as ten times the amount ordered.

> **2 mg**
>
> *not* **2.0 mg**

When the decimal point and zero following a whole number are dictated to emphasize the preciseness of a measurement, e.g., of a pathology specimen or a laboratory value, transcribe them as dictated. Do not, however, insert the decimal point and zero if they are not dictated.

> DICTATED & TRANSCRIBED
>
> **The specimen measured 4.8 × 2.0 × 3.4 mm.**
>
> *but*
>
> **The specimen measured 4.8 × 2 × 3.4 mm.**

For quantities less than 1, place a zero before the decimal point, except when the number could never equal 1 (e.g., in bullet calibers and in certain statistical expressions such as correlation coefficients and statistical probability).

> **0.75 mg**
> **.22-caliber rifle**

Do not exceed two places following the decimal except in special circumstances, e.g., specific gravity values, or when a precise measurement is intended. *See* nonmetric forms of measure *below.*

> **0.624 K-wire**
> **specific gravity 1.030**

Nonmetric forms of measure. Use the decimal form with nonmetric forms of measure when a precise measurement is intended and the fraction form would be both cumbersome and inexact. Two or more places may follow the decimal.

> **The 0.1816-inch screw was inserted.**

dollars and cents

Express exact amounts of dollars and cents with numerals, using a decimal point to separate dollars from cents.

> **$4.56**

When written out, lowercase all terms.

> **a million dollars**

Amounts less than $1. Use numerals; spell out and lowercase *cents.*

Do not use the decimal form. Do not use the dollar sign ($). Do not use the cent sign (¢) except in tabular matter.

> **8 cents *not* $.08 *not* 8¢**
> **20 cents *not* 20¢ *not* $.20**
> ***in tables:* 20¢ *not* .20¢ *not* $.20**

However, in tables that include amounts over $1, those amounts that are less than $1 should include a zero preceding the decimal so that entries are consistent.

> **$4.20**
> **$0.80**

Amounts over $1. Use the dollar sign ($) preceding the dollar amount, and separate dollars and cents by a decimal point.

Do not use a decimal following the dollar amount if cents are not included.

> **$1.08**
> **$1.20**
> **$40 *(Note: not $40.00, unless listed in a column with other amounts that include cents.)***

Subject-verb agreement. Monetary expressions take a singular verb when they are thought of as a sum, a plural verb when they are thought of as individual bills and coins.

> **A million dollars is a lot of money.**
> **The 50 quarters were stacked on the dresser.**

Ranges. Repeat the dollar sign or cent sign but do not repeat the word forms.

Use *to* instead of a hyphen with dollar-sign or cent-sign forms.

> **$4 to $5 *not* $4-$5**
> **10¢ to 15¢ *not* 10¢-l5¢**

Use *to* with word forms.

> **4 to 5 dollars *not* 4-5 dollars**
> **10 to 15 cents *not* 10-15 cents**

52

Possessive adjectives. Use *'s* or *s'*, whichever is appropriate, with units of money used as possessive adjectives.

> **1 dollar's worth**
> **2 cents' worth**

Do not use the possessive form with compound adjectives.

> **a 2-dollar bill**

International currencies. Sometimes it is important to distinguish US dollars from other currencies, such as Canadian dollars.

Note: There is no space between the letters and the $ symbol.

> **US$4.56**
> **Can$4.56**

Euro. The euro is the established (2002) currency for the European Union. Only time and usage will tell what the accepted plural forms will be. However, the official dossier from the European Union calls for the English plural of euro to be the same as the singular forms: *euro* and *cent*.

> **200 euro equal 200 cent**

The official abbreviation for the *euro* is EUR.

-hundreds

Numerals are preferred to words.

> **1900s** *not* **nineteen-hundreds**

fractions

Use numerals for fractional measurements preceding a noun. Join the fraction to the unit of measure with a hyphen, whether you use the symbol for the fraction or create it with whole numbers.

> **A ¼-inch incision was made.**
> **A 3/4-pound tumor was removed.**
> **The abdomen shows a 4-1/4-inch scar.**

Spell out fractional measurements that are less than one when they do not precede a noun.

> **The tumor weighed three quarters of a pound.**

Place a hyphen between numerator and denominator when neither contains a hyphen.

> **one-fourth empty**
> **two-thirds full**
>
> *but*
>
> **one forty-eighth *or* 1/48**
> **twenty-three thirty-eighths *or* 23/38**

Hyphenate fractions when they are written out and used as adjectives; do not hyphenate those written out and used as nouns.

> **one-half normal saline**
>
> **one third of the calf**
>
> **The patient cut the medication in half because she did not tolerate it well.**

midnight   Technically, the end of a day, not the beginning of a new one, so it is equivalent to 12 p.m. Do not capitalize. Do not use *12* with it.

> **Twin A was born at midnight, December 31, 2001; twin B at 12:14 a.m., January 1, 2002.**

number of   A collective noun that may be singular or plural. If preceded by *the*, it takes a singular verb. If preceded by *a*, it takes a plural verb.

> ***The* number of adhesions *was* minimal.**
>
> ***A* number of adhesions *were* present.**

HINT: *A number* = plural (nonspecific)
       The number = singular (specific)

Use *number* to refer to persons or things that can be counted. *Number* tells how many; *amount* tells how much (mass).

> **There was a small amount of bleeding, given the large number of wounds.**
>
> **A large number of people were present.**
>
> ***not* A large amount of people were present.**

No., #   Abbreviation and symbol for *number*. Note that the abbreviation capitalizes the initial letter and has an ending period: *No.* When the symbol # is used, the numeral follows it with no space between.

> **No. 4 blade**
> **#4 blade**
> **Tylenol No. 3**

Position or rank. Use the abbreviation or symbol with a figure to indicate position or rank.

> **He is No. 4 on the appointment list.**
>
> ***or* He is #4 on the appointment list.**

Model and serial numbers. Use the symbol with arabic numerals.

> **model #8546**
> **serial #185043**

Sizes of instruments or sutures. Do not use the abbreviation or symbol if "number" is not dictated. Either is acceptable (with the symbol preferred to the abbreviation) if "number" is dictated. Be consistent.

> **5-French catheter, #5-French catheter, No. 5-French catheter**
>
> **3-0 Vicryl, #3-0 Vicryl, No. 3-0 Vicryl**

Street addresses. Do not use the abbreviation or symbol before the number in street addresses.

> **166 Wallingford Avenue**
>
> *not* **No. 166 Wallingford Avenue**
>
> *not* **#166 Wallingford Avenue**

Suites, apartments, rooms. Use the abbreviation or symbol in suite, apartment, room, or similar number designations, when the noun designation is not used.

> **#104** *or* **No. 104** *or* **Apt. 104** *not* **Apt. #104**

Schools, fire companies, lodges. Do not use the abbreviation or symbol in names of schools, fire companies, lodges, or similar numbered units.

> **Public School 4**
> **Engine Company 3**

Page numbers. Lowercase *page* and use arabic numerals.

> **His history is detailed on page 2 of the report dated January 4, 2001.**

Lowercase roman numerals (i, v, x, etc.) refer to page numbers for preliminary material (contents pages, preface, etc.) in a book.

suture sizes

USP system. The United States Pharmacopeia system sizes, among other things, steel sutures and sutures of other materials. The sizes range from 11-0 (smallest) to 7 (largest). Thus, a size 7 suture is different from and larger than a size 7-0 suture.

Use 0 or 1-0 for single-aught suture; use the "digit hyphen zero" style to express sizes 2-0 through 11-0. Express sizes 1 through 7 with whole numbers. Place the symbol # before the size if "number" is dictated.

> **1-0 nylon** *or* **0 nylon**
> **2-0 nylon** *not* **00 nylon**
> **4-0 Vicryl** *not* **0000 Vicryl**
> **#7 cotton** *not* **0000000 cotton**
>
> DICTATED
> **3 and 4 oh silk**
>
> TRANSCRIBED
> **3-0 and 4-0 silk**

Brown and Sharp gauge (B&S gauge): System for sizing stainless steel sutures. Use whole arabic numerals ranging from 40 (smallest) to 20 (largest). Thus, a size 30 suture is smaller than a size 25.

telephone numbers

In a local seven-digit number, place a hyphen between the third and fourth digits. For phone numbers within the US, place a hyphen between the three-digit area code and the seven-digit telephone number. Alternatively, the area code may be placed in parentheses.

> **209-527-9620** *or* **(209) 527-9620**

International phone numbers require a country code, city code, and phone number. Dialing from the US, the international access code (011-) is also required, although it is not always written down.

NOTE: The use of periods or spaces in place of hyphens has long been the practice in other countries, and there is a trend toward this practice in the United States as well.

> 011-33-1-555-0864
> 011.33.1.555.0864

time

Abbreviations. Do not abbreviate English units of time except in virgule constructions and tables. Do not use periods with such abbreviations.

> **The patient is 5 days old.**
>
> **He will return in 3 weeks for followup.**
>
> **40 mm/h**

For on-the-hour expressions, it is preferable not to add the colon and 00. *See* military time *below*.

> **8:15 a.m.**
>
> *but* **8 a.m.** *or* **8 o'clock in the morning**
>
> *not* **8:00 a.m.,** *not* **8:00 o'clock**
>
> *not* **8 a.m. o'clock,** *not* **8 o'clock a.m.,** *not* **eight o'clock**
>
> **noon** *not* **12 o'clock**
>
> **midnight** *not* **12 o'clock**

Military time: Identifies the day's 24 hours by numerals 0100 through 2400, rather than 1 a.m. through noon and 1 p.m. through midnight.

Hours 0100 through 1200 are consistent with a.m. hours 1 through noon, while hours 1300 through 2400 correlate with p.m. hours 1 through midnight, respectively. This form always takes four numerals, so insert the preceding or following zeros as necessary. Do not separate hours from minutes with a colon. Do not use *a.m.* or *p.m.* If the word *hours* is not dictated it may be added for clarity, but this is not absolutely necessary.

> **1300 hours**
> **0845 hours**

Possessive adjectives. Use *'s* or *s'*, whichever is appropriate, with units of time used as possessive adjectives.

> **1 year's experience**
> **2 months' history**
> **3 days' time**

HINT: Any amount greater than 1 would require *s'*.

Time sequence. Give hours, minutes, seconds, tenths, and hundredths, in that sequence, using figures and colons as follows.

> **8:45:4.78**

Time span. Use hyphenated construction in a descriptive adjectival phrase expressing a time span.

> **1-month course**
> **3-day period**

Do not separate related time-span units by punctuation.

> **Labor lasted 8 hours 15 minutes.**

time zones   In extended forms, capitalize only those terms that are always capitalized, e.g., *Atlantic*, *Pacific*. Note: Some references capitalize *Eastern*, but some do not; be consistent. Lowercase *standard time* and *daylight time*. *Daylight time* is also known as *daylight-saving time*. Either form is correct, except that when linking the term to the name of a time zone, use *daylight time*, not *daylight-saving time*. Do not capitalize. Do not hyphenate.

> **Pacific daylight time**

Abbreviations. Use the abbreviation only when it accompanies a clock reading. Use all capitals in abbreviated forms, with noperiods. Do not use commas before or after the abbreviation.

> **10 a.m. EST**
> **Eastern standard time is...**

Event time. The time in the zone where an event occurs determines the date (and time) of the event.

tonight/
yesterday

Be specific when referring to dates. When *tonight* is dictated, include the date to which it refers except in direct quotations. Similarly, when *yesterday* is dictated, include the date to which it refers except in direct quotations.

> *The following was dictated on March 5, 2002:*
>
> DICTATED
> **The patient will be admitted to the hospital tonight.**
>
> TRANSCRIBED
> **The patient will be admitted to the hospital tonight, March 5, 2002.**

To avoid redundancy, do not combine the word *tonight* with the abbreviation *p.m.*

> **8 tonight** *or* **8 o'clock tonight** *or* **8:00 tonight** *or* **8 p.m.**
>
> *not* **8 p.m. tonight**

years

Use numerals to express specific years. When referring to a single year without the century, precede it by an apostrophe.

> **2001**
> **'99**

decades

Express with numerals except in special circumstances. Add *s* (without an apostrophe) to form the numeric plural.

> **The patient was well until the 1990s.**

Use a preceding apostrophe in shortened numeric expressions relating to decades of the century ('90s), but omit the preceding apostrophe in expressions relating to decades of age (80s).

> **He grew up in the '70s.**
> **He is in his 50s.**

Spell out and capitalize special references for decades.

> **the Roaring Twenties, the Gay Nineties**

centuries

Lowercase *century*. Spell out and lowercase century numbers *first* through *ninth*; use numerals for 10th and higher.

> **third century**
> **21st century**

Use a hyphen when *century* is part of a compound modifier.

> **20th-century music**

For proper names, use the form preferred by the organization.

> **The Twenty-First Century Foundation**
> **20th Century Fox**

The Final Word

The information provided in this chapter does not lend itself to a Quick Review study aid like some other chapters in this workbook do. The diverse nature of topics covered here would make it impossible to summarize these standards in a short list for quick study. Therefore, it will require you to work diligently through each topic, memorizing those standards that may be new or unfamiliar to you. This is a section where flash cards may also come in handy to assist you in keeping this information organized and less confusing. When transcribing, you should always consult a resource when you are unsure of the nature of the numeric referent you are hearing in dictation or how to apply a standard consistently.

Test Your Knowledge

Indicate the correct transcription of the following dictated excerpts in the space provided.

1. There was a two centimeter corneal abrasion at the two o'clock position.

_____

_____

_____

2. This is a five year old male who is brought to the ER by his mother.

_____

_____

_____

3. I last saw him on December 12th of 2004 and started him on Prevacid.

_____

_____

_____

4. She handed me two dollars worth of quarters in change.

_____

_____

_____

5. Upon admission, the child was given a half milligram of Cortisporin Otic to the right ear.

_____

_____

_____

6.   A number ten scalpel was used to incise the area.

_____

_____

_____

7.   The patient expired and was pronounced dead at
eighteen thirty-five.

_____

_____

_____

8.   The wound was closed using interrupted six oh nylon sutures.

_____

_____

_____

9.   We covered her with a tapering two week course of
steroids.

_____

_____

_____

10.   The patient was prescribed Lanoxin point oh five
milligrams.

_____

_____

_____

Test Your Knowledge

Answers

1. There was a 2 cm corneal abrasion at the 2 o'clock position.

2. This is a 5-year-old male who is brought to the ER by his mother.

3. I last saw him on December 12, 2004, and started him on Prevacid.

4. She handed me 2 dollars' worth of quarters in change.

5. Upon admission, the child was given 0.5 mg of Cortisporin Otic to the right ear.

6. A #10 scalpel was used to incise the area.

7. The patient expired and was pronounced dead at 1835. (*or* 1835 hours)

8. The wound was closed using interrupted 6-0 nylon sutures.

9. We covered her with a tapering 2-week course of steroids.

10. The patient was prescribed Lanoxin 0.05 mg.

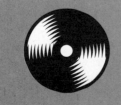

APPLICATION TEST
Take the application test for this chapter on your CD-ROM. Access the section for
Chapter 5: "Numeric Referents."

Percents, Proportions, Ranges, and Ratios

The diagnosis and management of disease is predicated upon scientific testing and measurement, the findings of which are expressed not only as singular values but often in contrast, comparison, or relationship to other closely related values. Examples of such expressions would be percents, proportions, ranges, and ratios. How does the MT determine the most appropriate way to represent this information in the record? This chapter will focus on special circumstances where numeric values might be expressed in terms of relationship to other values.

Going Deeper

For some determinations, a single value or finding is not as revealing or diagnostically helpful as the relationship between two or more values. In those instances, the significant finding may be derived from determining a proportion, ratio, or range. For example, high levels of low-density lipoprotein cholesterol (LDL-C) and low levels of high-density lipoprotein cholesterol (HDL-C) are significant independent positive risk factors for coronary artery disease and carotid artery atherosclerosis. Conversely, a high level of HDL-C is a significant independent negative risk factor. However, it is the total cholesterol (TC) to high-density lipoprotein cholesterol ratio that is a more valuable measure of coronary artery disease risk than TC or LDL-C levels alone. Similarly, the ratio of protein to creatinine in urine can be used to estimate the magnitude of proteinuria.[1]

An MT will also encounter references to percents as well as frequent references to the range between two values, the latter being quite common. Where ranges are concerned, there is often confusion about when to use the word *to* and when to use a hyphen between two numbers that describe a range of values. There are, as you will learn later in this chapter, specific criteria for when it is acceptable to utilize a hyphen and when the word *to* must be used.

Significant laboratory values and many medication dosages often involve expressions of proportion. References to the liquid delivery form of a medication will often include a reference to the strength of that medication per usual dose—per milliliter (mL) for injectables and drops and per 5 mL or 15 mL for oral liquids and syrups.[2] It is thus not uncommon to hear a physician dictate an ear drop, for example, by both strength and dosage: "Otomycin 10,000 units per milliliter, one drop in each ear twice a day."

These numeric expressions, like others covered to this point, represent areas of critical content in a patient record and potential for misinterpretation and clinical error. Knowledge of the clinical context will help guide you in applying these standards. Knowing whether the dictated phrase "two to three" should be expressed as *2 to 3, 2-3,* or *2:3* will depend entirely on the MT's awareness of the context in which this phrase is dictated and whether a range or ratio is being referenced. Thus, care will need to be taken to ensure that they are expressed accurately and without ambiguity.

Rules & Exceptions

over, virgule   Use a virgule (/) to express *over* or *on a scale of* in expressions such as the following.

> DICTATED
> **blood pressure 160 over 100**
> **reflexes 2+ out of 4**
> **grade one over four murmur**
> **grade two to three over six murmur**

> **TRANSCRIBED**
> **blood pressure 160/100**
> **reflexes 2+/4**
> **grade 1/4 murmur**
> **grade 2/6 to 3/6 murmur**
> *or* **grade 2 to 3 over 6 murmur**

percent

Note that *percent* is a single word (not *per cent*). Do not use the abbreviation *pct.* except in tables. Instead, use % or *percent*.

> **50% *or* fifty percent *not* 50 pct.**

Use the symbol % after a numeral. Do not space between the numeral and the symbol.

> **13% monos, 1% bands**
>
> **She has had a 10% increase in weight since her last visit.**
>
> **MCHC 34%**
>
> **10% solution**

Use numerals for the number preceding %.

> **50% *not* fifty %**

When the number is written out, as at the beginning of a sentence, write out *percent*.

> **Fifty percent of the patients were given a placebo.**

According to the SI (International System of Units), it is common and acceptable for percents to be expressed as a fraction of one. MT experience would indicate that it is more common and acceptable for *percent* to be dropped in dictation (and thus in transcription). Use the expression dictated; do not convert.

> **polys 58%** *or* **polys 0.58** *or* **polys 58**
>
> **MCHC 34%** *or* **MCHC 0.34** *or* **MCHC 34**

In a range of values, repeat % (or *percent*) with each quantity.

> **Values ranged from 13% to 18%.**
> *not* **Values ranged from 13 to 18%.**
>
> **Fifty percent to eighty percent...**
> *not* **Fifty to eighty percent...**

Less than 1 percent. When the amount is less than 1 percent, place a zero before the decimal.

> **0.5%** *not* **.5%**

With whole numbers, avoid following the number by a decimal point and a zero, since such forms are easily misread. The decimal point and zero may be used if it is important to express exactness. Use it if dictated. (Note: Keep in mind the dangerous abbreviations recommendations about leading and trailing zeros.)

> **5%** *not* **5.0%**

Use decimals, not fractions, with percents.

> **0.5%** *not* **1/2%**

proportions   Always use numerals in expressions of proportions.

> **5 parts dextrose to 1 part water**

range   Use numerals. It is acceptable to use a hyphen between the limits of a range if the following five conditions are met:

1. The phrases "from...to," "from...through," "between...and" are **not** used.

2. Decimals and/or commas do not appear in the numeric values.

3. Neither value contains four or more digits.

4. Neither value is negative.

5. Neither value is accompanied by a symbol.

When all five conditions are met, a hyphen may be used. (*To* may be used instead, even when the conditions are met).

> **Our new office hours will be 1-4 p.m. Tuesdays and Thursdays.**
>
> **8-12 wbc** *or* **8 to 12 wbc**

When any of the five above conditions is **not** met, use *to* (or other appropriate wording) in place of a hyphen.

> **3+ to 4+ edema** *not* **3-4+ edema**
> **$4 to $5 million**
> **-25 to +48**
>
> **Weight fluctuated between 120 and 130 pounds**
> **Platelet counts were 120,000 to 160,000.**

Do not use a colon between the limits of a range. Colons are used to express ratios, not ranges.

> **80-125** *not* **80:125**

Blood pressure ranges should be expressed consistently, using *to* or a hyphen between the ranges of the diastolic pressures and systolic pressures, but these should not be combined in a virgule (/) construction as they may be misunderstood.

> DICTATED
> **Blood pressure was 100 to 120 over 70 to 80.**

> TRANSCRIBED
> **Blood pressure was 100-120 over 70-80.**
> *or* **Blood pressure was …100 to 120 over 70 to 80.**
> *or* **Blood pressure was in the 100-120 over 70-80 range.**
>
> **Not acceptable because they may be misunderstood are:**
> **100-120/70-80** *and* **100/70 to 120/80**

For EKG sequential leads: Repeat the *V*. Do not use a hyphen or dash.

> **leads V1 through V5** *or* **leads V$_1$ through V$_5$**
> *not* **V1 through 5** *or* **V$_1$ through $_5$**
> *not* **V1-V5** *or* **V$_1$-V$_5$**
> *not* **V1-5** *or* **V$_{1-5}$**

For ranges related to money: Repeat the dollar sign or cent sign but do not repeat the word forms. Use *to* instead of a hyphen with dollar-sign or cent-sign forms.

> **$4 to $5** *not* **$4-$5**
> **10¢ to 15¢** *not* **10¢-15¢**

Intravertebral disk space. Use a hyphen to express the space between two vertebrae (the intervertebral space). It is not necessary to repeat the same letter before the second vertebra, but it may be transcribed if dictated.

> **C1-2** *or* **C1-C2**
> **L5-S1**

In a range of values, repeat % (or *percent*) with each quantity. (See section on *percent* on p. 95.)

ratio   The relationship of one quantity to another. Express the value with the numerals separated by a colon. Do not replace the colon with a virgule, dash, hyphen, or other mark.

Mycoplasma 1:2

cold agglutinins 1:4

Zolyse 1:10,000

Xylocaine with epinephrine 1:200,000

Use *to* or a hyphen instead of a colon when the expression includes words or letters instead of values. Consult appropriate references for guidance.

I-to-E ratio

Myeloid-erythroid ratio

FEV-FVC ratio

QUICK REVIEW

1. Use a virgule (/) to express *over* or *on a scale of* or *out of.*

2. In a range of values, repeat the virgule (/) for each value expressed. Do not combine.

3. For percent, use the symbol (%) when used with a numeral. Spell out *percent* when the number it accompanies is spelled out.

4. In a range of values, repeat the percent (%) for each value expressed. Do not combine.

5. Do use a leading zero for amounts less than one percent. Do not use a trailing zero after whole number amounts.

6. Use decimals, not fractions, with percents.

7. Always use numerals in expressions of proportions.

8. Always use numerals to express a range. Do not use a hyphen in a range expression unless all five conditions listed in this chapter have been met.

9. Express blood pressure ranges consistently; use a hyphen or *to* between diastolic value ranges and between systolic value ranges. Do not combine those value ranges in a virgule (/) construction, however.

10. For EKG leads, repeat the V, and do not use a hyphen or dash in a range expression.

11. Use a hyphen between two vertebrae to express an interverte-bral disk space.

12. Use a colon (:) to express a ratio value where numerals are used.

13. Use a hyphen or the word *to* when expressing a ratio where words are used.

The Final Word

The concepts expressed in this chapter relate to value expressions that, when transcribed correctly, will demonstrate your commitment to a high-quality document. Expressing ratios and proportions correctly and understanding and applying the rules related to ranges, while less important where clinical accuracy is concerned, are demonstrable evidence of your understanding of transcription standards. Clinical accuracy, of course, leaves off at the point where all of the health encounter information is recorded accurately. But quality picks up at that point and concerns itself in the way that information is expressed. These are standards of style that speak to the readability of the document and its ability to communicate information in a clear, clean, and concise manner.

Test Your Knowledge

Indicate the correct transcription of the following dictated excerpts in the space provided.

1. The patient's blood pressure was in the seventy to eighty over one-twenty range.

2. I told her those side effects occurred in only two to five percent of patients.

3. He was treated with Epinal point five percent drops to both eyes.

4. We instilled epinephrine one to ten thousand into the area of the incision.

5. Ferritin normal value ranges for women are between eighteen and one-sixty nanograms per milliliter.

6. She was given half percent Isopto Carpine drops for her glaucoma.

_____

_____

_____

7. The patient had an FEV to FVC of sixty-five percent.

_____

_____

_____

8. There was some depression in leads V one through V six.

_____

_____

_____

9. VITAL SIGNS: Blood pressure eighty to ninety over one-thirty to one-forty.

_____

_____

_____

10. Fifty percent of his patients are from the inner city.

_____

_____

_____

Test Your Knowledge

Answers

---

1. The patient's blood pressure was in the 70 to 80 over 120 range. *or* The patient's blood pressure was in the 70-80 over 120 range. *or* The patient's blood pressure was in the 70/120 to 80/120 range.

---

2. I told her those side effects occurred in only 2% to 5% of patients.

---

3. She was treated with Epinal 0.5% drops to both eyes.

---

4. We instilled epinephrine 1:10,000 into the area of the incision.

---

5. Ferritin normal value ranges for women are between 18 and 160 ng/mL.

---

6. She was given 0.5% Isopto Carpine drops for her glaucoma.

---

7. The patient had an FEV:FVC of 65%.

---

8. There was depression in leads V1 through V6.

---

9. VITAL SIGNS: Blood pressure 80-90 over 130-140. *or* VITAL SIGNS: Blood pressure 80 to 90 over 130 to 140.

---

10. Fifty percent of his patients are from the inner city. *(correct as is)*

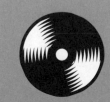

APPLICATION TEST
Take the application test for this chapter on your CD-ROM. Access the section for
Chapter 6: "Percents, Proportions, Ranges, and Ratios."

References

1. Beers, Mark H., and Berkow, Robert, editors. *The Merck Manual of Geriatrics, 3rd edition*. Whitehouse Station, NJ: Merck Research Laboratories, 2000.

2. Drake, Randy, and Drake, Ellen. *Saunders Pharmaceutical Word Book 2005*. Philadelphia, PA: W.B. Saunders, 2005.

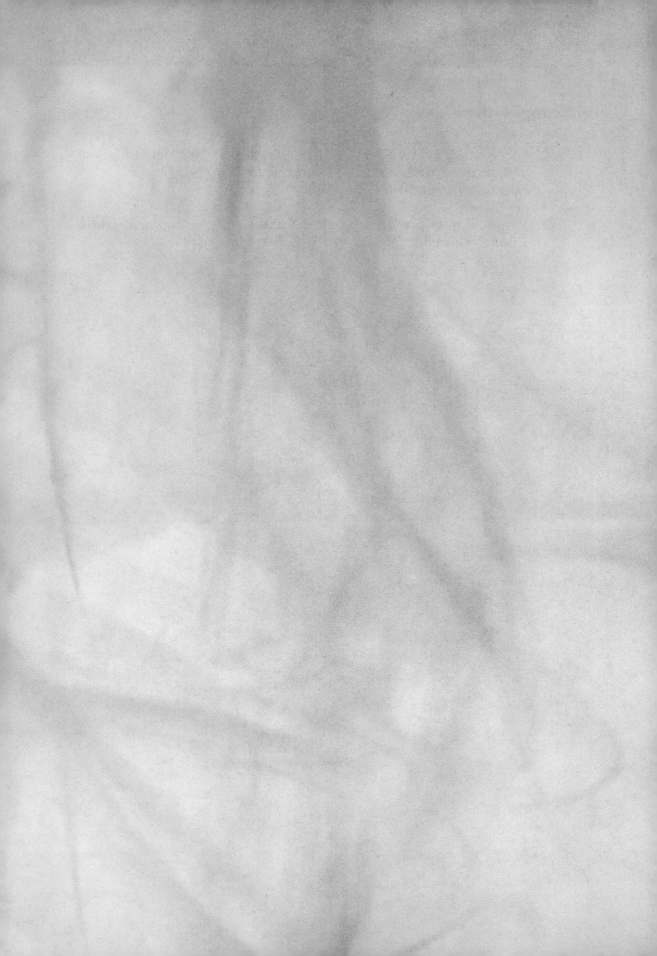

Qualifiers

Units of Measure
Rules and Exceptions

BOS Statement

Where?
BOS pp. 214–222

The International System of Units (Système International d'Unités, abbreviated SI) is the system of metric measurements adopted in 1960 at the Eleventh General Conference on Weights and Measures of the International Organization for Standards.

Since the 1977 recommendation of the 30th World Health Assembly that SI units be used in medicine, some medical journals use the SI to a limited degree, some use it only in conjunction with conventional units, and some have not yet adopted it.

The adoption of SI in the documentation of patient care is likewise sporadic, but it is sufficiently widespread, in whole or in part, to warrant the attention of medical transcriptionists. It should be noted that, although some units from the apothecary system remain in use, all elements of the apothecary system have been dropped from the compendium of the United States Pharmacopeia (USP) system.

Additionally, the accelerated movement toward international adoption of the electronic patient record is likely to strengthen the adoption of the SI in order to facilitate communication across borders.

Going Deeper

The previous unit focused on the delineation of *quantity* in the medical record, those critical value areas of a report where numbers, or fractions thereof, are used to quantify certain measurements in a patient's diagnosis, treatment, and care. This unit, however, will focus on those common terms that *qualify* that information. This chapter will outline the most common and significant qualifiers in the medical record—*units of measure*. These two sides of the same coin are equally important in providing a full diagnostic picture. In order for a patient's diagnostic information to be meaningful, it must be quantified and qualified. A numeric value alone will be of little significance without an understanding of the method or measurement from which that value is derived or the system by which it is being measured. If I tell you that a patient's wound measurement was an 8, that information alone would be insufficient. *Is it 8 inches? 8 cm? 8 fingerbreadths?* The value must be qualified. Likewise, a general measurement of "a few inches" does not provide the diagnostic context that is often critical to care. The value must be more clearly quantified. A quantified numeric value and a qualified unit of measure will provide the greatest level of detail, and it is this kind of data that is extracted for patient care and for statistical warehousing.

Most values in the record must be qualified for them to have meaning, although quite often the qualifier is implied. While it will be important for you to memorize and recognize the myriad units of measure that are commonly encountered in dictation, you will not be required in most settings to provide these units where they are not dictated. In the laboratory section of the report, for example, it is common practice for physicians to dictate just the name of a particular test and its numeric value, though virtually all of those values have a corresponding unit of measure that can be verified in a reputable laboratory resource. There are some facilities that do require their transcriptionists to include the units of measure with each laboratory value, whether dictated or not; however, this scenario is rare and is not common practice.

Memorizing the abbreviations for these units of measure will be the most important aspect of this section. A dictator will rarely, if ever, dictate the unit of measure in its abbreviated form. A physician will not say that the patient was given "50 M G of Tylenol." Rather, he will dictate that the patient was given "50 milligrams of Tylenol," and the MT will be expected to abbreviate those units appropriately.

If you recall from Chapter 1, this was one of the exceptions to the rule for not expanding abbreviations dictated in full:

> **Terms dictated in full.** Do not use an abbreviation when a term is dictated in full.
>
> **Exception:** Units of measure (milligrams, centimeters, etc.).

The Metric System   One of the complex aspects of this particular chapter is the contradiction that can be found in some areas between what is identified in the International System of Units, what is identified as part of the metric system, and what is commonly encountered in transcription. It will be important to understand that the SI system is an evolved metric system that is now being widely adopted worldwide. There is still some inconsistency, however, in whether a value is reported in older metric units or the new SI units, though most units are similar. In addition, transcriptionists in the US will also find that old Imperial units and apothecary units are still used in certain areas of our healthcare system. This, of course, will come as no surprise to any American MT student who has likely grown up with the reality that the United States has not fully adopted the metric system. Our healthcare documentation is a reflection of this reality. In any given patient record, you will find references that range from older apothecary units (*drops, drams*) to English units (*pounds, ounces, feet*) to metric units (*mg, cm, mL*). Fortunately, these occur consistently in their contexts, at least within the US healthcare system. Height and weight, for example, are always dictated in English units, while the weight of the organs in an autopsy or pathology report is usually reported and recorded in metric units. Fortunately, the transcriptionist is rarely ever left wondering which unit is being referred to and will likely not encounter a flip-flop in usage in these areas. The only exception to this, of course, will be for MTs who transcribe in countries where the metric system may be more widely utilized. A transcriptionist transcribing for Canadian facilities will encounter some differences in style there and will probably encounter metric measurements virtually everywhere in a report. If those same transcriptionists perform work for US healthcare providers, however, they may find themselves hearing different units being dictated in the same contexts.

While all sections in the BOS related to the International System of Units or metric system have been included in this text, you will want to pay close attention to those sections where the BOS clearly indicates that the standard of practice in the industry may not comply with the SI information being provided. There are few areas where this contradiction is encountered, but it is important to make note of them.

Rules & Exceptions

International System of Units

basic units and properties of the SI

Major characteristics of the SI are decimals, a system of prefixes, and a standard defined as an invariable physical measure.

base unit	SI symbol	basic property
meter	m	length
kilogram	kg	mass
second	s	time
ampere	A	electric current
kelvin	K	thermodynamic temperature
candela	cd	luminous intensity
mole	mol	amount of substance

Two supplementary units of the SI are:

radian	**rad**	**plane angle**
steradian	**sr**	**solid angle**

units derived from SI's basic units

derived unit	name and symbol	basic unit derived from
area	square meter (m^2)	meter
volume	cubic meter (m^3)	meter
frequency	hertz (Hz)	kilogram
pressure	pascal (Pa)	kilogram
force	newton (N)	kilogram
density	kilogram per cubic meter (kg/m^3)	kilogram

speed, velocity	meter per second (m/s)	meter
acceleration	meter per second squared (m/s^2)	meter
electric field strength	volt per meter (V/m)	meter

NOTE: Hertz, pascal, and newton are eponyms but are not capitalized when they are spelled out, even when they stand alone unaccompanied by a numeric value.

prefixes and symbols

The SI combines prefixes with the basic units to express multiples and submultiples of those units. Factors are powers of 10. Note that the SI refers to shortened forms of measure as symbols, not abbreviations.

factor	prefix	symbol
10^{24}	yotta-	y
10^{21}	zetta-	z
10^{18}	exa-	E
10^{15}	peta-	P
10^{12}	tera-	T
10^{9}	giga-	G
10^{6}	mega-	M
10^{3}	kilo-	k
10^{0}	hecto-	h
10	deca-	da
10^{-1}	deci-	d
10^{-2}	centi-	c
10^{-3}	milli-	m
10^{-6}	micro-	mi
10^{-9}	nano-	n
10^{-12}	pico-	P
10^{-15}	femto-	f
10^{-18}	atto-	a
10^{-21}	zepto-	Z
10^{-24}	yoctu-	Y

According to the *AMA Manual of Style*, exponents that are multiples of 3 are recommended, and those prefixes that are not multiples of 3 (e.g., hecto-, deca-, deci-, and centi-) are to be avoided in scientific writing. That avoidance obviously does not extend to patient records, as evidenced by MTs' frequent encounters with the prefix centi- (centimeter, centigrade, centigray) and occasional encounters with deci- (decigram, deciliter).

In general, medical transcriptionists should apply the following rules and guidelines for the SI, but this is not always possible. Exceptions that are necessary, logical, or commonly accepted in medical transcription are noted.

abbreviations   Abbreviate most units of measure that accompany numerals and include virgule constructions. Use the same abbreviation for singular and plural forms. Do not use periods with abbreviated units of measure.

> **1 g**
> **20 g**
> **40 mm/h**

The following are abbreviations for the metric units of measure most commonly used in medical reports. Do not use periods.

cm	**centimeter**
dL	**deciliter**
g	**gram**
L	**liter**
mEq	**milliequivalent**
mg	**milligram**
mL	**milliliter**
mm	**millimeter**
mmHg	**millimeter of mercury**
mmol	**millimole**
msec, ms	**millisecond**

Use these abbreviations only when a numeric quantity precedes the unit of measure. Do not add an *s* to indicate plural form. Do not capitalize most metric units of measure or their abbreviations. Learn the obvious exceptions, and consult appropriate references for guidance.

cm	**centimeter**
dB	**decibel**
Hz	**hertz**
L	**liter**

Use the decimal form with metric units of measure even when dictated as fractions, unless they are not easily converted.

DICTATED
four and a half millimeters

TRANSCRIBED
4.5 mm *not* **4-1/2 mm**

DICTATED
four and a third millimeters

TRANSCRIBED
4-1/3 mm

area, volume, and magnification

The SI uses the multiplication sign in expressions of area, volume, and magnification. In medical transcription, use a lowercase *x* for area and volume; space before and after it to enhance readability.

2 x 2 mm area

Magnification is generally expressed with a capital *X* (although a lowercase *x* is acceptable), placed before the size of magnification, without a space.

X30 magnification

commas	Drop the comma in numbers of four digits. In numbers of five or more digits, the SI replaces the comma with a half space. This is not always possible in medical transcription, nor is it commonly seen in healthcare records, so the continued use of the comma is acceptable and preferred in numbers of five or more digits in medical transcription. Do conform to the SI rule eliminating both the comma and the half space in numbers that contain decimal points.

> **1234**
>
> **12,345**
>
> **12345.67**

decimals v fractions	Use the decimal form of numbers when a fraction is given with an abbreviated unit of measure or for a precise measurement. Use mixed fractions for approximate measurements; these often represent time.

> **4.5 mm**
>
> **5-1/2 days** *or* **5½ days**
>
> **3-3/4 hours**

drug dosages	It is anticipated that all drug dosages will eventually be expressed in SI units.
exponents	When technology does not readily allow exponents to be expressed as superscripts, abbreviations like *cu* and *sq* are acceptable. Do not place the exponent numerals on the line in these expressions as they are not easily read when expressed in this manner.

> **10^5** *or* **10 to the 5th**
>
> **3 m^2** *or* **3 sq m** (*not* m2)
>
> **9 m^3** *or* **9 cu m** (*not* m3)

numerals	Use arabic numerals for all quantities with units of measure. Place a space between the numeral and the symbol for the unit of measure. Exceptions: Do not place a space between the numeral and the percent sign, the degree sign, or the Celsius (or Fahrenheit) symbol.

Place the quantity and the unit of measure on the same line of text; where possible, do not allow one line of text to end with the quantity and the next line to begin with the unit of measure.

> **48 kg**
>
> **13.5 mm**
>
> **48%**
>
> **40°C**

When a number and unit of measure begin a sentence, consider recasting the sentence so as to avoid beginning it with a numeral and unit of measure. Otherwise, write out both the number and unit of measure.

> DICTATED
> **Twenty milliequivalents of KCl was given.**
>
> TRANSCRIBED
> **KCl 20 mEq was given.**
>
> *or*
>
> **Twenty milliequivalents of KCl was given.**

percentage values

According to the SI, it is common and acceptable for percentage values to be expressed as a fraction of one. MT experience would indicate that it is more common and acceptable for percent to be dropped in dictation (and thus in transcription). Use the expression dictated. Do not convert unless the forms are mixed; then make them consistent.

> **polys 58%** *or* **polys 0.58** *or* **polys 58**
> **MCHC 34%** *or* **MCHC 0.34** *or* **MCHC 34**

rad v gray; calorie v joule

The SI converts rad to gray (Gy) and calorie to joule. Transcribe as dictated; do not make the conversion unless directed to do so.

units of time and time abbreviations

Do not abbreviate expressions of English units of time except in virgule constructions. Do not use periods with such abbreviations. Note: In pharmaceutical expressions such as q.h. and q.i.d., the terms are Latin (h., hora; d., die) and require periods for clarity.

minute	min
week	wk
month	mo
hour	h
day	d
year	y

The patient is 5 days old.

He will return in 1 week for followup.

40 mm/h

q.4 h.

Efforts have been made here to extract the basic applications of SI rules and guidelines to medical transcription. As indicated, SI usage affects or is affected by many other areas of medical transcription style and practice: grammar, abbreviations, numerals, punctuation, plurals, etc.

More detail about the SI and SI units is available from the *AMA Manual of Style*, from which much of the above information was drawn, but keep in mind that the AMA text speaks to the preparation of medical manuscripts for publication and does not address the preparation of medical reports, i.e., the communication of patient information through medical dictation and transcription. As indicated, some of the differences are pronounced.

Nonmetric Units of Measure

Spell out common nonmetric units of measure (ounce, pound, inch, foot, yard, mile, etc.) to express weight, depth, distance, height, length, and width, except in tables. Do not use an apostrophe or quotation marks to indicate feet or inches, respectively (except in tables).

> **4 pounds**
>
> **5 ounces**
>
> **14 inches**
>
> **5 feet**
>
> **5 feet 3 inches** *not* **5′ 3″** *not* **5 ft. 3 in.**

Do not abbreviate most nonmetric units of measure, except in tables. Use the same abbreviation for both singular and plural forms; do not add *s*.

> **5 in. (***use* **in.** *only in a table***)**

Do not use a comma or other punctuation between units of the same dimension.

> **The infant weighed 5 pounds 3 ounces.**
>
> **He is 5 feet 4 inches tall.**

Use a hyphen to join a number and a unit of measure when they are used as an adjective preceding a noun.

> **5-inch wound**
>
> **8-pound 5-ounce baby girl**

Temperature, Temperature Scales

degrees

Express temperature degrees with numerals except for zero.

> **zero degrees**
>
> **36 degrees**
>
> **36°C**

Use *minus* (not the symbol) to indicate temperatures below zero.

> **minus 48°C**

If the temperature scale name (Celsius, Fahrenheit, Kelvin) or abbreviation (C, F, K) is not dictated, it is not necessary to insert it.

> **38°C** *or* **38 degrees Celsius** *or* **38 degrees**

Use the degree symbol (°) if available, immediately followed by the abbreviation for the temperature scale. If the degree symbol is not available, write out degrees (and the temperature scale name, if dictated). Note: There is no space between the degree symbol and the abbreviation for the temperature scale.

> **98°F** *or* **98 degrees Fahrenheit**

Celsius

Metric-system temperature scale, designed by and named for Celsius, a Swedish astronomer. Also known as *centigrade scale*, but *Celsius* is the preferred term. Normal human temperature on the Celsius scale is 36.7°, often rounded to 37°. In the Celsius system, zero degrees represents the freezing point of water; 100 degrees represents the boiling point at sea level.

Abbreviation: C (no period).

> **37°C**
>
> *or* **37 degrees Celsius**

Fahrenheit

Temperature scale designed by and named for Fahrenheit, a German-born physicist who also invented the mercury thermometer. Normal human temperature on the Fahrenheit scale is 98.6°.

Abbreviation: F (no period).

> **96.5°F**
>
> *or* **96.5 degrees Fahrenheit**

Kelvin

Temperature scale based on Celsius but not identical. Used to record extremely high and low temperatures in science. The starting point is zero, representing total absence of heat and equal to minus 273.15 degrees Celsius. To convert to Kelvin from Celsius, subtract 273.15 from the Celsius temperature.

Abbreviation: K (no period).

Capitalize *Kelvin* in references to the temperature scale, but lowercase *kelvin* when referring to the SI temperature unit. The abbreviation is always capitalized.

73

The Final Word

Taking the time to memorize the many units of measure covered in this chapter will be a wise investment of time as you move into consistent daily transcription. These are terms you will hear frequently, often in every record you encounter. Some units of measure, like those specific to radiation and nuclear medicine, will be encountered less often or only if you find yourself consistently transcribing in that specialty environment. For the MT who anticipates a career in acute care transcription, however, being familiar with all of these units will be very important.

It may also be helpful when memorizing these units to mentally categorize them by measurement type so that their application in a clinical context will make more sense to you. Knowing that an injectable medication could only be measured in liquid units will predispose you to interpreting those units accurately and *not* using a measurement for length (mm) when a measurement for liquid (mL) is indicated in context. The Quick Review section below should assist you in beginning to group these units together according to type.

QUICK REVIEW 1: UNITS BY TYPE

* Note: A number of units have been added to this chart and are not found in the BOS sections above. Many of these will also be encountered in transcription.

Basic Property	Metric or SI Units	Non-Metric Units
length	meter (m)	fingerbreadth, inch, feet, yard, mile
mass	gram (g)	ounce, pound
time	second (s), minute (m)	
electrical current	ampere (A)	
electrical voltage	volts (V)	
electrical resistance	ohms	
temperature	degrees Celsius (C) kelvin (K)	degrees Fahrenheit (F)
luminous intensity	candela (cd)	
amount of substance	mole (mol)	
area	square meter (m^2)	square inch, square yard
volume	cubic meter (m^3)	cubic inch, cubic yard
frequency	hertz (Hz)	
energy, work	joule (J)	
pressure	pascal (Pa)	pounds per square inch (psi)
force	Newton (N)	
density	kilogram per cubic meter (kg/m^3)	pounds per cubic foot
speed, velocity	meter per second (m/s)	feet per second
acceleration	meter per second squared (m/s^2)	feet per second squared
electric field strength	volt per meter (V/m)	
radiation	milliCuries (mCi)	

QUICK REVIEW 2: COMMON PREFIXES

PREFIX	FRACTIONAL UNIT
deci-	one-tenth
centi-	one-hundredth
milli-	one-thousandth
micro-	one-millionth
nano-	one-billionth
pico-	one-trillionth
deka-	10 units
hecto-	100 units
kilo-	1000 units
mega-	one million units
giga-	one billion units
tera-	one trillion units

QUICK REVIEW 3: METRIC UNITS MOST COMMONLY USED IN MEDICAL REPORTS

ABBREVIATION	UNIT
cm	centimeter
dL	deciliter
g	gram
L	liter
mEq	milliequivalent
mg	milligram
mL	milliliter
mm	millimeter
mmHg	millimeters of mercury
mmol	millimole
msec, ms	millisecond

Test Your Knowledge

I. For each of the units below, provide the correct abbreviation.

√**1.** decibel _____

√**2.** hertz _____

3. joule _____

4. ampere _____

5. microgram _____

6. millisecond _____

7. nanomole _____

8. kilograms _____

√**9.** centimeter _____

10. radian _____

√**11.** milligram _____

√**12.** deciliter _____

13. kelvin _____

14. cubic meter _____

15. liter _____

16. Celsius _____

17. milliequivalent _____

18. nanoseconds _____

√**19.** gram _____

20. square meters _____

II. Transcribe the following dictated excerpts in the space provided.

1. The patient was cooled to twenty-eight degrees Celsius on cardiopulmonary bypass.

_____
_____
_____

2. Defibrillator threshold measurements were one point one milliamperes and six hundred ohms of resistance with a sixteen millivolt R wave and a zero point six volt threshold.

_____
_____
_____

3. Doppler studies revealed a regurgitant jet across the mitral valve, with a jet velocity of four point two five meters per second and a gradient of seventy-two millimeters of mercury.

_____
_____
_____

4. A ten millimeter trocar was introduced and advanced without difficulty.

_____
_____
_____

5. The proximal portion of the colon was characterized by the presence of multiple nodular areas averaging from three to five millimeters in diameter.

_____
_____
_____

6.   The dosage is two hundred twenty-five milligrams per meter squared of Taxol and carboplatin.

_____

_____

_____

7.   On physical examination, her weight is two hundred three pounds, height five feet three inches, and BSA one point nine five meters squared.

_____

_____

_____

8.   The patient has already received two grams of Rocephin that would provide coverage for the next twenty-four hours.

_____

_____

_____

9.   Cerebral activity over the left side consisted of high-amplitude, poorly sustained four to five Hertz waveforms.

_____

_____

_____

10.   POSTOPERATIVE DIAGNOSIS: Missed abortion at five and a half weeks.

_____

_____

_____

Test Your Knowledge

Answers

I.

1. dB		**11.** mg
2. Hz		**12.** dL
3. J		**13.** K
4. A		**14.** m^3
5. mcg		**15.** L
6. msec *or* ms		**16.** C
7. nmol		**17.** mEq
8. kg		**18.** nsec *or* ns
9. cm		**19.** g
10. rad		**20.** m^2

II.

1. The patient was cooled to 28 degrees Celsius on cardiopulmonary bypass. *or* The patient was cooled to 28°C on cardiopulmonary bypass.

2. Defibrillator threshold measurements were 1.1 mA and 600 ohms of resistance with a 16 mV R wave and a 0.6-V threshold.

3. Doppler studies revealed a regurgitant jet across the mitral valve, with a jet velocity of 4.25 m/sec (*or* m/s) and a gradient of 72 mmHg.

4. A 10 mm trocar was introduced and advanced without difficulty.

5. The proximal portion of the colon was characterized by the presence of multiple nodular areas averaging from 3-5 (*or* 3 to 5) mm in diameter.

6. The dosage is 225 mg/m^2 of Taxol and carboplatin.

7. On physical examination, her weight is 203 pounds, height 5 feet 3 inches, and BSA 1.95 m^2.

8. The patient has already received 2 g of Rocephin that would provide coverage for the next 24 hours.

9. Cerebral activity over the left side consisted of high-amplitude, poorly sustained 4-5 (*or* 4 to 5) Hz waveforms.

10. POSTOPERATIVE DIAGNOSIS: Missed abortion at 5½ weeks.

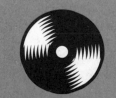

APPLICATION TEST
Take the application test for this chapter on your CD-ROM. Access the section for
Chapter 7: "Units of Measure."

Drug Terminology & Chemical Nomenclature

8

As far back as ancient times, healers and physicians have turned to pharmacology to treat symptoms and cure disease. No generation, however, has witnessed a greater evolution, application, and use of drugs than our current one. Although there is a growing trend in medicine to seek alternative remedies, most of these are still based on herbal pharmacology, and despite the emergence of these new remedies, traditional medicine is still by far the treatment of choice in the U.S. healthcare system.

The application of medicinal remedies in the management and treatment of disease is a core component of patient care and, thus, a critical presence in documentation. As a student of medical transcription, you will likely study pharmacology as a separate course component and become familiar with the types, classifications, descriptions, and applications of core drug groups. In addition, you will be expected to recognize many commonly prescribed drugs by specialty and use. In this chapter, we will explore the standards of style related to the transcription of drug terminology and chemical nomenclature. Both entail some very specific rules for *how* this information should be represented in writing, and as always, the focus is on clarity of communication in the record.

Going Deeper

It is important to keep in mind that pharmacology is based on fundamental chemistry. For those who have never had a course in chemistry, much of this may be new and unfamiliar. This chapter will walk you through some of the common chemical elements that you will encounter in transcription. Most of these elements are found either in the human body, in large quantities or trace amounts, or in the drugs formulated to cure and/or manage disease. How these elements bond with each other to form a compound as well as how they interact with each other both outside and within the human body can be critical to the predication of a drug's efficacy *and* the potential harm or benefit that drug may have on a patient. Likewise, the balance of the basic elements in the human body is critical to homeostasis, or physical wellbeing, so these chemical references form the basis of most laboratory testing and evaluation as well.

Rules & Exceptions

Chemical Nomenclature

elements and symbols

Names of elements are not capitalized. The symbols for chemical elements always include an initial capital letter; if there is a second letter, it is always lowercase. Never use periods or other punctuation with chemical symbols.

The following is a list of some of the more commonly encountered elements from the periodic table, with their symbols.

barium	Ba
calcium	Ca
carbon	C
cesium	Cs
chlorine	Cl
cobalt	Co
copper	Cu
gadolinium	Gd
gallium	Ga
gold	Au

hydrogen	H
iodine	I
iron	Fe
lead	Pb
magnesium	Mg
mercury	Hg
nitrogen	N
oxygen	O
potassium	K
silver	Ag
sodium	Na
sulfur	S
technetium	Tc
zinc	Zn

compounds   Lowercase the names of chemical compounds written in full.

Never use hyphens in chemical elements or compounds, whether used as nouns or adjectives. Note: Some *isotopes* are joined to the chemical name with a hyphen; refer to an appropriate drug resource for verification.

**carbon dioxide
potassium
carbon monoxide poisoning**

**chemical
names**   Do not capitalize chemical names, except at the beginning of a sentence.

acetylsalicylic acid

oxygen

concentration   Use brackets to express chemical concentration. When concentrations are expressed as percentages, use the percent sign rather than the spelled-out form, and do not use brackets.

$[HCO_3^-]$ *or* **$[HCO3^-]$**

15% HNO_3 *or* **$HNO3$**

formulas

Use parentheses for innermost units, adding brackets, then braces, if necessary. (Note that this is different from regular text, which uses brackets for the innermost parenthetical insertion and parentheses for the outermost.) Italics may also be used for some portions; consult chemistry references. Two examples of chemical formulas follow.

chlorphenoxamine hydrochloride

2-[1-(4-chlorophenyl)-1-phenylethoxy]-N,N-dimethylethanamine hydrochloride

hydroxychloroquine sulfate

7-chloro-4-{4-[ethyl(2-hydroxyethyl)amino]-1-methylbutylamino}-quinoline sulfate

biochemical terminology

Write out biochemical terms in healthcare documents because their abbreviations may not be readily recognized by healthcare professionals.

Use abbreviated forms only in tables and in communications among biochemical specialists.

The following are examples of biochemical groups, terms, and abbreviations (3-letter and/or 1-letter).

amino acids of proteins

phenylalanine	Phe, F
proline	Pro, P
tryptophan	Trp, W

bases and nucleosides

cytosine	Cyt
purine	Pur
uracil	Ura

common ribonucleosides

adenosine	Ado, A
cytidine	Cyd, C
uridine	Urd, U

sugars and carbohydrates	
fructose	Fru
glucose	Rib

Drug Terminology

abbreviations and punctuation

Use lowercase abbreviations with periods for Latin abbreviations that are related to doses and dosages. Do not use abbreviations found on the "Dangerous Abbreviations" list from the Institute for Safe Medication Practices.

Avoid using all capitals because they emphasize the abbreviation rather than the drug name. Avoid lowercase abbreviations without periods because some may be misread as words.

Do not translate.

abbreviation	Latin phrase	English translation
a.c.	ante cibum	before food
b.i.d.	bis in die	twice a day
gtt.	guttae	drops (better to spell out drops)
n.p.o.	nil per os	nothing by mouth
n.r.	non repetatur	do not repeat
p.c.	post cibum	after food
p.o.	per os	by mouth
p.r.n.	pro re nata	as needed
q.4 h.	quaque 4 hora	every 4 hours
q.h.	quaque hora	every hour
q.i.d.	quater in die	4 times a day
t.i.d.	ter in die	3 times a day
u.d.	ut dictum	as directed

NOTE: We have inserted a space after the numeral *4* in *q.4 h.* on the advice of the ISMP so that the number is more easily and clearly read.

Invalid Latin abbreviations such as *q.a.m. (every morning)* and mixed Latin and English abbreviations such as *q.4 hours (every 4 hours)* have become commonplace. However, as with all abbreviations, avoid those that are obscure (like *a.c.b.* for *before breakfast*) or dangerous. For example, *b.i.w.* is both obscure **and** dangerous. It is intended to mean *twice weekly* but it could be mistaken for *twice daily*, resulting in a dosage frequency seven times that intended.

It is acceptable to express a range in dosage times in abbreviated format.

> **q.2-3 h.**
> **q.4-6 h.**

NOTE: AAMT continues to discourage dropping periods in lowercase abbreviations that might be misread as words (for example, *bid* and *tid*). If you must drop the periods, use all capitals, but keep in mind that the overuse of capitals, particularly in relation to drug doses and dosages, would draw more attention to the capitalized abbreviations than to the drug names themselves.

Do not use commas to separate drug names from doses and instructions. In a series of drugs for each of which the dose and/or instructions are given, use commas to separate each complete entry. Exception: Use semicolons or periods when entries in the series have internal commas. Medications may also be listed vertically.

> **The patient was discharged on Coumadin 10 mg daily.**
>
> **The patient was discharged on Carafate 1 g q.i.d., 40 minutes after meals and at bedtime; bethanechol 25 mg p.o. q.i.d.; and Reglan 5 mg at bedtime on a trial basis.**
>
> **He was sent home on Biaxin 500 mg b.i.d., Atrovent inhaler 2 puffs q.i.d., and Altace 5 mg daily.**
>
> **CURRENT MEDICATIONS**
> **1. Lescol 2 mg at bedtime.**
> **2. DiaBeta 5 mg 1 q.a.m.**
> **3. Aspirin 325 mg 1 daily.**
> **4. Xanax 0.25 mg t.i.d. p.r.n.**

dose and dosage

Dose means *the amount to be administered at one time*, or *total amount administered*.

Dosage means *regimen* and is usually expressed as a quantity per unit of time.

dose	**5 mg**
dosage	**5 mg q.i.d.**

Oral dosage forms include pills, tablets, and capsules. Liquid dosage forms may be solutions, emulsions, and suspensions. Topical dosage forms include suspensions or emulsions, such as ointments, creams, lotions, and gels. Other dosage forms include granules, powders, transdermal patches, ocular inserts, suppositories, subdermal pellets, solutions, sprays, drops, and injections.

The most common dosage route is oral for absorption through stomach or intestinal walls. Another common route is parenteral, such as intravenous, intramuscular, subcutaneous, intra-arterial, intradermal, intrathecal, and epidural. Other routes include topical, inhalation, rectal, vaginal, urethral, intramedullary, ocular, nasal, sublingual, and otic.

systems of measurement for drugs

Most pharmaceutical measurements for weight and volume are in the metric system. Although some units from the apothecary and avoirdupois systems remain in use, it should be noted that all elements of the apothecary system have been dropped from the compendium of the United States Pharmacopeia system (USP).

apothecary system

weight	liquid measure
1 grain (gr)	1 minim
1 scruple (20 gr)	1 fluidram (60 minims)
1 dram (60 gr)	1 fluidounce (8 fluidrams)
1 ounce (480 gr)	1 pint (16 fluidounces)
1 pound (5760 gr)	1 gallon (4 quarts or 8 pints)

Note: Either fluidounce or fluid ounce is an acceptable spelling.

> **avoirdupois system**
>
> 1 grain
> 1 ounce (437.5 grains)
> 1 pound (16 ounces or 7000 grains)

brand name, trade name, trademark

The brand name is the manufacturer's name for a drug; it is the same as the trade name, trademark, or proprietary name. It may suggest a use or indication, and it often incorporates the manufacturer's name.

Capitalize brand names, trade names, and trademark names.

> **Tagamet**
> **Bayer**

Use of idiosyncratic capitalization is optional.

> **pHisoHex** *or* **Phisohex**

The trade name is a broader term than trademark, identifying the manufacturer but not the product.

Capitalize trade names.

> **Dr. Scholl's**

code name

The code name is the temporary designation for an as-yet-unnamed drug; it is assigned by the manufacturer. It may include a code number or code designation (number-letter combination).

chemical name

The chemical name describes the chemical structure of a drug. The American Chemical Society, which is the internationally recognized source for such names, follows a set of guidelines established by chemists.

Do not capitalize chemical names.

> **acetylsalicylic acid**

generic name

The generic name is also known as the nonproprietary name, the established, official name for a drug. In the United States, it is created by the US Adopted Names Council (USAN). International nomenclature is coordinated by the World Health Organization.

Generic names are in the public domain; their use is unrestricted.

Do not capitalize generic names. When the generic name and brand name of a medication sound alike, use the generic spelling unless it is certain that the brand name is being referenced.

> **aminophylline *(generic name)***
> *not* **Aminophyllin *(brand name)***

isotope nomenclature

Used in reference to radioactive drugs.

When the element name, not the symbol, is used, place the isotope number on the line after the name in the same font and type size; do not superscript or subscript. Space between the element name and the isotope number. Do not hyphenate either the noun or the adjectival form.

> **iodine 128**
> **technetium 99m**

When the element symbol is used, place the isotope number as a superscript immediately before the symbol. Alternatively, use the following format: element symbol, space (*not* hyphen), isotope number (on the line), *or* avoid the nonsuperscript form by using the element name followed by the isotope number.

> ^{128}**I** *or* **I 128** *or* **iodine 128**
> ^{99m}**Tc** *or* **Tc 99m** *or* **technetium 99m**

For trademarked isotopes, follow the style of the manufacturer. In trademarks, the isotope is usually joined to the rest of the name by a hyphen; it may or may not be preceded by the element symbol.

> **Glofil-125**
> **Hippuran I 131**

interferons

A small class of glycoproteins that exert antiviral activity.

Use nonproprietary names as discussed below. For trade names and additional guidance, consult the USAN dictionary or other appropriate reference.

For general classes of compounds or single compounds, follow the lowercase interferon by the spelled-out Greek letter; use the Greek symbol in abbreviations. Note: *alfa* is the correct spelling in these terms, not *alpha*.

> **interferon alfa   IFN-α**
> **interferon beta   IFN-β**
> **interferon gamma IFN-γ**

For individual, pure, identifiable compounds with nonproprietary names, add a hyphen, an arabic numeral, and a lowercase letter.

> **interferon alfa-2a**
> **interferon alfa-2b**
> **interferon gamma-1a**
> **interferon gamma-1b**

For names of mixtures of interferons from natural sources, add a hyphen, a lowercase *n*, and an arabic numeral.

> **interferon alfa-n1**
> **interferon alfa-n2**

multiple-drug regimens

Abbreviations for multiple-drug regimens are acceptable if widely used and readily recognized.

> **MOPP (methotrexate, vincristine sulfate, prednisone, and procarbazine)**

vitamins

Lowercase *vitamin*, capitalize the letter designation, and use arabic numerals (in subscript form if available). Do not use a hyphen or space between the letter and numeral.

> **vitamin B12** *or* **vitamin B$_{12}$**
> **B12 vitamin** *or* **B$_{12}$ vitamin**

vitamin	drug name
vitamin B1	thiamine hydrochloride
vitamin B2	riboflavin
vitamin B6	pyridoxine hydrochloride
vitamin B12	cyanocobalamin
vitamin C	ascorbic acid
vitamin D2	ergocalciferol
vitamin D3	cholecalciferol
vitamin K1	phytonadione
vitamin K3	menadione

The Final Word

Some of the chemical references covered in this chapter are rather obscure and rarely encountered. Certainly, you will not likely be asked to transcribe chemical formulas in mainstream patient documentation. You may, however, find yourself employed or contracted by a physician or practice that is involved in research, case studies, and clinical trials, the documentation of which is critical for publication. It is not uncommon for an MT to transcribe this ancillary kind of documentation in those settings. You may, then, encounter more detailed scientific data and references to chemical formulas and processes that you would not typically find in patient records. In the instance of research being documented for formal publication in a medical journal, understanding the appropriate style for transcribing that data will be very valuable to the MT in that setting and an asset to the physician(s) in that practice.

What is essential in this chapter, of course, is the information related to transcribing drug dose and dosage information, including the myriad abbreviations that identify frequency and application. These you will transcribe consistently from chart to chart, so this is an area you should pay particular attention to. Memorize the Latin abbreviations in particular so that their transcription becomes second nature to you.

Test Your Knowledge

I. For each of the phrases below, provide the correct Latin abbreviation.

1. twice a day _____   **6.** after food _____

2. as directed _____   **7.** four times a day _____

3. every hour _____   **8.** before food _____

4. nothing by mouth _____   **9.** by mouth _____

5. do not repeat _____   **10.** every four hours _____

II. Each sentence below contains at least one error in transcribing information covered in this chapter. Correct the sentences in the space below.

1. He was sent home on erythromycin 500 mg Q.I.D., Theo-Dur 300 mg B.I.D. and Tenormin 50 mg Q.D.

_____

_____

_____

2. She is given 12 Thorazine 25 mg suppositories to use 1 or 2 q.6 hours prn.

_____

_____

_____

3.   Serum vitamin-B12 level was 598, well within normal limits.

_____

_____

_____

4.   On her last visit she was begun on Nifedipine 20 mg PO and I will increase this to 30 mg.

_____

_____

_____

5.   We first injected 5.17 mCi of TC-99M intravenously.

_____

_____

_____

6.   The patient will be given Actimmune, an interferon gamma 1-B, for her CGD.

_____

_____

_____

7.   Laboratory tests indicated significant anemia, so we have given her 10,000 units of Epoetin alpha.

_____

_____

_____

8.   She was given KCL 20 mEq q.i.d.

_____

_____

_____

9. Initial electrolytes revealed Sodium 130, Potassium 4, Chloride 99, and Bicarbonate 12.

_____

_____

_____

10. He will follow up with me q.weekly until this resolves.

_____

_____

_____

Test Your Knowledge

Answers

I.

1. b.i.d.

2. u.d.

3. q.h.

4. n.p.o.

5. n.r.

6. p.c.

7. q.i.d.

8. a.c.

9. p.o.

10. q.4 h.

II.

1. He was sent home on erythromycin 500 mg q.i.d., Theo-Dur 300 mg b.i.d. and Tenormin 50 mg q.d.

2. She is given 12 Thorazine 25 mg suppositories to use 1 or 2 q.6 h. p.r.n.

3. Serum vitamin B12 (*or* B_{12}) level was 598, well within normal limits.

4. On her last visit she was begun on nifedipine 20 mg p.o. and I will increase this to 30 mg.

5. We first injected 5.17 mCi of Tc 99m (*or* ^{99m}Tc) intravenously.

6. The patient will be given Actimmune, an interferon gamma-1b, for her CGD.

7. Laboratory tests indicated significant anemia, so we have given her 10,000 units of epoetin alfa.

8. She was given KCl 20 mEq q.i.d.

9. Initial electrolytes revealed sodium 130, potassium 4, chloride 99, and bicarbonate 12.

10. He will follow up with me weekly (*or* every week) until this resolves.

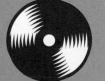

APPLICATION TEST
Take the application test for this chapter on your CD-ROM.
Access the section for
Chapter 8: "Drug Terminology & Chemical Nomenclature."

Classifications

The diagnostic process is rarely simple. While there are a great many conditions that can be singularly described, others are far more complex, necessitating identification of not only the condition or disease but also its stage in evolution or development. Even something as straightforward as a fracture must be identified by type, location, and remodeling stage. Certainly, most chronic diseases and cancers by nature require close monitoring and determination of progress or status. To say that someone has a tumor of the brain is not sufficiently diagnostic for effective treatment planning. The oncologist must also determine the type, size, location, aggressive nature, rate of growth, and potential metastasis of that tumor to best treat the disease and manage its potential course. Similarly, an orthopedist might need to describe a broken bone as more than just a fracture. Its location, type, and severity are also critical to determining immediate treatment and long-term care.

Care providers obviously can use long lists of adjectives to describe things like tumors and fractures, but they often find it more efficient to incorporate these descriptions into a single abbreviated lexicon, or naming system, that can quickly identify the condition, disease, or physical assessment. For example, a physician may dictate that a newborn infant had Apgar scores of 9 and 10. Since the Apgar system is used worldwide, anyone who encounters this in the record understands that at 1 and 5 minutes after birth, the newborn's pulse, breathing, color, tone, and reflex irritability were rated on a scale of 0 to 2. There is no need to delineate these individually or describe the Apgar process. This is much more efficient and consistently communicative than a rambling narrative outlining the patient's pulse, breathing, color, etc. Only when one of these is grossly abnormal would we see a physician deviate from a straightforward Apgar score to a notation of the specific findings.

Classification systems and terms are frequently used to identify and define conditions, and each system has a specific method for classifying and expressing those values. Some are expressed with arabic numbers and some are expressed with roman numerals. Some are so organized that specific expressions may require a blend of numbers and letters, both uppercase and lowercase, some with hyphens and some without. Each classification system is unique, and there will be no quick and easy method for determining what these are. You will simply need to understand and memorize each one.

Going Deeper

Keep in mind that classifications systems exist for the purposes of organization and standardization. Type 2 diabetes mellitus, for example, correlates to a specific set of identifiers and parameters that are understood and recognized by any healthcare facility or healthcare provider. This common identifying language facilitates continuity of care across a spectrum of delivery points. The same is true for all other classification definitions and systems you will encounter in this chapter. Many of them, you will note, are specialty specific and arise out of a common desire among the practitioners of that specialty to adopt a language that is universal across the delivery spectrum. This facilitates not only care but also the exchange of data and research between specialty providers when addressing these conditions and diseases. If each psychiatrist had a unique and proprietary system for assessing depression, for example, then none of the data gathered by one psychiatrist would correlate with the data gathered by another. It would be very difficult to compare apples with apples, so to speak.

You will encounter a variety of terms associated with classification: *grade*, *stage*, *type*, *class*, *level*, *score*, *degree*, *criteria*, *scale*, *system*, and *status*. Some are preceded by their value; others precede the value. Some have accompanying units or symbols (like % for the Rule of Nines – See pp. 152–153). Again, each one is unique and requires both understanding and memorization to ensure appropriate transcription of classifications and their accompanying values when encountered in dictation.

Because there are so many classifications specific to cancer staging and grading, those classification systems will be covered specifically in Chapter 15. All other classification terms and systems identified in the *BOS* are outlined below.

Rules & Exceptions

Classification Systems

Where?
BOS p. 71

BOS Statement

Some classification systems use arabic numerals and others call for roman. In some systems there is no agreement on the use of roman versus arabic numerals. There is a trend away from the use of roman numerals, and generally speaking, the preference is for using arabic numerals unless it is documented that roman numerals are required. Many classification systems are listed below; check appropriate references for additional guidance.

Apgar score   Assessment of newborn's condition in which pulse, breathing, color, tone, and reflex irritability are each rated 0, 1, or 2, at one minute and five minutes after birth. Each set of ratings is totaled, and both totals are reported. Named after Virginia Apgar, MD. Do not confuse with APGAR questionnaire for family assessment. Use initial capital only. Express ratings with arabic numerals. Write out the numbers related to minutes, so that attention is drawn to the scores and confusion is avoided.

> **Apgars 7 and 9 at one and five minutes.**

Ballard scale A scoring system for assessing the gestational age of infants based on neuromuscular and physical maturity. Scores are converted to gestational age (in weeks). Express in arabic numerals.

score	age (weeks)
5	26
10	28
15	30
20	32
25	34
30	36
35	38
40	40
45	42
50	44

blood groups Use single or dual letters, sometimes with a subscript letter or number. If subscripts are not available, place the numeral immediately following and on the line with the letter.

> **group A**
> **group A_1 *or* group A1**
> **group A_1B *or* group A1B**

burn classifications Burns are described as 1st, 2nd, 3rd, and 4th degree, according to burn depth. AAMT recommends dropping the hyphen in the adjective form (e.g., 1st degree burn), though use of the hyphen is acceptable. Expressing ordinals as numerals is preferred to writing them out: 1st, 2nd, 3rd, and 4th degree burns, *not* first, second, third, and fourth degree burns.

Rule of Nines: Formula, based on multiples of 9, for determining percentage of burned body surface. This formula does not apply to children because a child's head is disproportionately large.

head	9%
each arm	9%
each leg	18%
anterior trunk	18%
posterior trunk	18%
perineum	1%

Berkow formula: Rule of Nines adjusted for a patient's age. Assigns a higher percentage to a child's head, which is larger than an adult's head in proportion to its body.

Catterall hip score

Rating system for Legg-Perthes disease (pediatric avascular necrosis of the femoral head).

Use roman numerals I (no findings) through IV (involvement of entire femoral head).

Child classification of hepatic risk criteria

Classification of operative risk.

Capitalize *Child* (eponymic term), lowercase *class*, and capitalize the letter that follows.

> **Child class A**
> **Child class B**
> **Child class C**

Crowe classification

System for classifying developmental dysplasia of the hip.

grade I	less than 50% subluxation
grade II	50% to 75% subluxation
grade III	75% to 100% subluxation

decubitus ulcers

Decubitus ulcers are classified using roman numerals from stage I (nonblanchable erythema of intact skin) through stage IV (full-thickness skin loss with extensive tissue destruction).

diabetes mellitus classifications

The following information on the classification of diabetes mellitus is taken from the "Report of the Expert Committee on the Diagnosis and Classification of Diabetes Mellitus," first published in 1997 and further modified since then (available through the American Diabetes Association, www.diabetes.org). The two major changes made by the Expert Committee that affect medical transcriptionists are as follows:

1. The move away from the terms insulin-dependent diabetes and non-insulin-dependent diabetes. The report stressed that patients with any form of diabetes may require insulin at some stage of their disease but that such use of insulin does not, of itself, classify the disease.

2. The use of arabic rather than roman numerals for diabetes types.

type 1 and type 2 diabetes

The Expert Committee adopted the use of arabic numerals for diabetes types in order to improve communication, stating that it is too easy to confuse the roman numeral II for the arabic number 11.

Type 1 diabetes (formerly type I, insulin-dependent, or juvenile-onset diabetes).

Type 2 diabetes (formerly type II, non-insulin-dependent, or adult-onset diabetes).

The third class of diabetes comprises eight types and encompasses more than 45 specific diseases.

The fourth class is gestational diabetes mellitus (GDM), defined as any degree of glucose intolerance with its onset or first recognition during pregnancy. Classifications of diabetes mellitus in pregnancy include:

class A: (gestational diabetes): Transient.

class B: Initial onset after age 20, less than 10 years' duration, controlled by diet. Patient may become insulin-dependent during pregnancy but not need insulin after delivery.

class C: Onset between ages 10 and 19. Insulin-dependent patient will need increased insulin during pregnancy but will likely return to pre-pregnancy dosage after delivery.

class D: Onset before age 10, with more than 20 years' duration. Patient has hypertension, diabetic retinopathy, and peripheral vascular disease.

class E: Patient has calcification of pelvic vessels.

class F: Patient has diabetic nephropathy.

Infants of diabetic mothers may be described as

- LGA infants: large for gestational age. Infants of class A, B, and C mothers are apt to be LGA.

- SGA infants: small for gestational age. Infants of class D, E, and F mothers are apt to be SGA.

Epworth Sleepiness Scale

Measures daytime sleepiness on a scale of 1 to 24. Use arabic numerals.

Less than 8: Normal sleep function

8-10: Mild sleepiness

11-15: Moderate sleepiness

16-20: Severe sleepiness

21-24: Excessive sleepiness

> **The patient's Epworth Sleepiness Scale is 16.**

fracture classification systems

Garden: Subcapital fractures of femoral neck.

Lowercase stage and use arabic numerals: stage 1 (incomplete) through stage 3 (most complete).

LeFort: Classification of facial fractures.

Use roman numeral I, II, or III. Do not space between *Le* and *Fort*.

> **LeFort I**

Mayo: Classification of olecranon fractures. Use roman numerals and capital letters.

type	description
I	undisplaced
IA	noncomminuted
IB	comminuted
II	displaced, stable
IIA	noncomminuted
IIB	comminuted
III	displaced, unstable
IIIA	noncomminuted
IIIB	comminuted

Neer-Horowitz: Classification of proximal humeral physeal fractures in children. Use roman numerals I (less than 5 mm displacement) through IV (displaced more than two-thirds the width of the shaft).

> **Neer-Horowitz II**

Salter: Classification of epiphyseal fractures. Use roman numerals I (least severe) through VI (most severe).

> **Salter III fracture**

Schatzker: Classification of tibial plateau fractures in terms of injury and therapeutic requirements. Lowercase *type* and use roman numerals: type I (least complicated) through type VI (most complicated).

Salter-Harris: Fracture involving the physis in children. Use roman numerals I (fracture across the physis only) through V (crush injury to physis).

> **Salter-Harris fracture type II.**

stress fractures: Lowercase *grade* and use roman numerals I (local symptoms, negative radiographs, positive bone scan) through IV (local symptoms, actual bone fracture identified on radiographs, positive bone scan).

Note: A grade 0 indicates an asymptomatic patient with negative radiographs and negative bone scan.

French scale   Sizing system for catheters, sounds, and other tubular instruments. Each unit is approximately 0.33 mm in diameter. Express in arabic numerals. Precede by # or No. if the word "number" is dictated. Do not lowercase *French*.

> **5-French catheter**
> **#5-French catheter**
> **5F catheter (note: according to Dorland's & Stedman's)**
> **catheter, size 5 French**

Keep in mind that *French* is linked to diameter size and is not the eponymic name of an instrument. Thus, it is a 15-French catheter, *not* a French catheter, size 15.

GAF scale   Global Assessment of Functioning. A scale used by mental health professionals to assess an individual's overall psychological functioning. Typically reported in a psychiatric diagnosis as axis V. Use arabic numerals 0 (inadequate information) through 100 (superior functioning in a wide range of activities).

> **Axis V GAF = 60; flat affect.**

GARF scale   Global assessment of relational functioning. This scale is used by mental health professionals to measure an overall functioning of a family or other ongoing relationship. Use arabic numerals from 0 (inadequate information) to 100 (relational unit functioning satisfactorily from self-report of participants and from perspectives of observers).

Glasgow coma scale   Describes level of consciousness of patients with head injuries by testing the patient's ability to respond to verbal, motor, and sensory stimulation.

Each parameter is scored on a scale of 1 through 5, and then totals are added together to indicate level of consciousness. (Glasgow refers to Glasgow, Scotland.)

score	level of consciousness
14 or 15	normal
7 or less	coma
3 or less	brain death

GVHD grading system
Graft-versus-host disease. Use arabic numerals 1 (mild) through 4 (severe), placed on the line directly after the abbreviation (no space). May also be expressed as clinical grade 1 through 4.

GVHD1 *or* GVHD clinical grade 1

GVHD2 *or* GVHD clinical grade 2

GVHD3 *or* GVHD clinical grade 3

GVHD4 *or* GVHD clinical grade 4

Harvard criteria for brain death
In addition to body temperature equal to or higher than 32°C and the absence of central nervous system depressants, all of the following criteria must be met in order to establish brain death.

unreceptivity and unresponsiveness

no movement or breathing

no reflexes

flat electroencephalogram (confirmatory)

Hunt and Hess neurological classification
Classifies prognosis of patients with hemorrhage. Write out and lowercase *grade*; do not abbreviate. Use arabic numerals 1 through 4.

grade 3

Kurtzke disability score

Two-part scoring system to evaluate patients with multiple sclerosis. Part one evaluates functional systems (pyramidal, cerebellar, brain stem, sensory, bowel and bladder, visual, mental, and other). Part two is a disability status scale from 0 to 10. Use arabic numerals.

magnitude scale

Measures earthquake magnitude. A one-unit increase on the scale equals a tenfold increase in ground motion. Express with arabic numerals and decimal point.

> **She was injured in an earthquake measuring 6.6 magnitude.**

Mallampati-Samsoon classification of airway

With the patient seated upright, mouth opened as wide as possible and tongue protruding, the anesthesiologist examines the airway—soft palate, tonsillar fauces, tonsillar pillars, and uvula—to evaluate the ease or difficulty of intubation: class I (easy intubation) through class IV (nearly impossible intubation). Lowercase *class* and use roman numerals.

NOTE: There is an increasing trend for anesthesiologists, pulmonologists, and laryngologists to refer to this simply as a "Mallampati class" or a "Mallampati airway."

Neer staging

System for classifying shoulder impingement.

stage	description
I	inflammation and edema of the rotator cuff
II	degenerative fibrosis
III	partial or full-thickness tear

NYHA classification of cardiac failure

Widely adopted classification of cardiac failure that was developed by the New York Heart Association. Lowercase *class*; use roman numerals I through IV.

I	asymptomatic
II	comfortable at rest, symptomatic with normal activity
III	comfortable at rest, symptomatic with less than normal activity
IV	severe cardiac failure, symptomatic at rest

> DIAGNOSIS
> **Cardiac failure, class III.**

Outerbridge scale

Assesses damage in chondromalacia patellae. Lower case *grade*. Use arabic numerals 1 (minimal) through 4 (excessive).

> DIAGNOSIS
> **Chondromalacia patellae, grade 3.**

physical status classification

A classification developed by the American Society of Anesthesiologists to classify a patient's risk of complications from surgery. Lowercase class and use arabic numerals (1 through 5). The capital letter E is added to indicate an emergency operation.

> **class 1E**

psychiatric diagnoses

A multiaxial system is often used in diagnosing psychiatric patients. Axis I is for all psychiatric disorders except mood disorders and mental retardation; axis II is for all personality disorders and mental retardation; axis III is for general medical conditions; axis IV, psychosocial and environmental problems; and axis V is an assessment of function, usually using the global assessment of functioning (GAF) scale. The following example demonstrates a typical psychiatric diagnosis along with the applicable diagnostic codes found in the *Diagnostic and Statistical Manual of Mental Disorders, 4th edition* (DSM-IV), which are consistent with ICD-9-CM and ICD-10 codes.

Axis I	296.2	Major depressive disorder, single episode, severe, without psychotic features.
	305.0	Alcohol abuse.
Axis II	301.6	Dependent personality disorder.
Axis III		None.
Axis IV		Threat of job loss.
Axis V		GAF = 3 (current).

Rancho Los Amigos cognitive function scale
Neurologic assessment tool. Levels I through VIII are written with roman numerals.

I	no response
II	generalized response to stimulation
III	localized response to stimuli
IV	confused and agitated behavior
V	confused with inappropriate behavior (nonagitated)
VI	confused but appropriate behavior
VII	automatic and appropriate behavior
VIII	purposeful and appropriate behavior

SOFAS
Social and Occupational Functioning Assessment Scale. The SOFAS is an instrument used by mental health professionals to assess an individual's social and occupational functioning only. Use arabic numerals from 0 (inadequate information) through 100 (superior functioning in a wide range of activities).

TIMI system
Thrombolysis in myocardial infarction. A grading system (grade 0 to 3) for coronary perfusion; evaluates reperfusion achieved by thrombolytic therapy. Lowercase grade and use arabic numerals.

> **The patient had TIMI grade 3 flow at 90 minutes following thrombolytic therapy.**

trauma score
Scoring system that measures systolic blood pressure, respiratory rate and expansion, capillary refill, eye opening, and verbal and motor responses on a scale of 2 through 16. Score predicts injury severity and probability of survival. Use arabic numerals.

The Final Word

It certainly would be easier on the medical transcriptionist if a single naming and classification structure were used to identify these conditions and diseases, but these classification systems are developed autonomously and have very little correlation with each other. However, there are some commonalities that can be identified. You will note that most fracture classifications, for example, use roman numerals to describe the complexity or severity of the fracture type. Undoubtedly, as new fracture types were identified, there was a tendency to adopt the same kind of expression already seen with other fracture classifications. Most of the systems outlined above, however, do not correlate to each other and each has a unique method of identification. Your study for this section will need to focus on *what* disease or condition these systems identify and *how* they are recorded.

It should be noted that the evolution of both the electronic health record and database-driven documentation systems is likely to necessitate some changes in the standards above. There is a growing trend to replace all roman numeral indicators with arabic numbers for the purposes of clarity and electronic document management. We may see a preference for the single character "3" where the roman numeral "III" has previously been the standard, but only time will tell. Future updates of the *Book of Style* will likely address the impact of the EHR on these and other standards.

QUICK REVIEW

Roman Numerals	Arabic Numbers
Catterall score (I-IV)	Apgar score (8-10)
Crowe classification (grade I-III)	Ballard scale (5-50)
Decubitus ulcers (stage I-IV)	burns (1st-4th degree)
LeFort fractures (I-III)	Rule of Nines (%)
Neer-Horowitz fractures (I-IV)	Diabetes mellitus (type 1 and 2)
Salter fractures (I-VI)	Epworth Sleepiness Scale (1-24)
Schatzker fractures (I-VI)	Garden fractures (stage 1-3)
Salter-Harris fractures (I-V)	French scale for catheters
stress fractures (grade 0-IV)	GAF scale (0-100)
Mallampati-Samsoon airway (class I-IV)	GARF scale (0-100)
Neer staging (stage I-III)	Glasgow coma scale (1-15)
NYHA cardiac failure (class I-IV)	GVHD system (clinical grade 1-4)
Psychiatric diagnosis (Axis I-V)	Hunt and Hess (grade 1-4)
Ranchos Los Amigos cognitive function (level I-VIII)	Kurtzke disability score, part 2 (0-10)
	Outerbridge scale (grade 1-4)
	physical status (class 1-5)
	SOFAS (0-100)
	TIMI system (grade 0-3)
	trauma score (2-16)

Letters	
(A, B, C etc.)	**Combination**
Child class (A, B, C)	Blood groups (A1B)
Gestational diabetes (class A-F)	Mayo fractures (I, IA, IB…IIIB)

Test Your Knowledge

I. Match the disease or condition on the left with the name of its classification system on the right.

1. dysplasia of the hip _____ A. Catterall

2. multiple sclerosis _____ B. LeFort

3. facial fractures _____ C. Mallampati-Samsoon

4. sleepiness _____ D. Glasgow

5. operative risk _____ E. Ballard

6. epiphyseal fractures _____ F. Crowe

7. airway _____ G. Epworth

8. tibial plateau fractures _____ H. Garden

9. level of consciousness _____ I. Hunt and Hess

10. femoral neck fractures _____ J. Kurtzke

11. chondromalacia patellae _____ K. Child

12. brain hemorrhage _____ L. Salter

13. gestational age _____ M. Mayo

14. olecranon fractures _____ N. Outerbridge

15. Legg-Perthes disease _____ O. Schatzker

II. Provide a description of how each classification system indicated below should be expressed in transcription.

Example: Outerbridge scale Arabic numbers, grade 1-4

1. Apgar score _____

2. LeFort fractures _____

3. Crowe classification _____

4. GAF scale _____

5. psychiatric diagnosis _____

6. Catterall score _____

7. Epworth scale _____

8. Mallampati-Samsoon _____

9. Ballard scale _____

10. NYHA classification of cardiac failure _____

11. decubitus ulcers _____

12. SOFAS _____

13. Neer-Horowitz fractures _____

14. Glasgow coma scale _____

15. Child class _____

Test Your Knowledge

Answers

I.

1.	F	**9.**	D
2.	J	**10.**	H
3.	B	**11.**	N
4.	G	**12.**	I
5.	K	**13.**	E
6.	L	**14.**	M
7.	C	**15.**	A
8.	O		

II.

1. Arabic numbers from 8 to 10

2. Roman numerals from I to III

3. Roman numerals; *grade* I to III

4. Arabic numbers from 0 to 100

5. Roman numerals; *Axis* I to IV

6. Roman numerals from I to IV

7. Arabic numbers from 1 to 24

8. Roman numerals; *class* I to IV

9. Arabic numbers from 5 to 50

10. Roman numerals; *class* I to IV

11. Roman numerals; *stage* I to IV

12. Arabic numbers from 0 to 100

13. Roman numerals from I to IV

14. Arabic numbers from 1 to 15

15. Capital letters from A to C

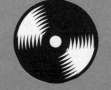

APPLICATION TEST
Take the application test for this chapter on your CD-ROM.
Access the section for
Chapter 9: "Classifications."

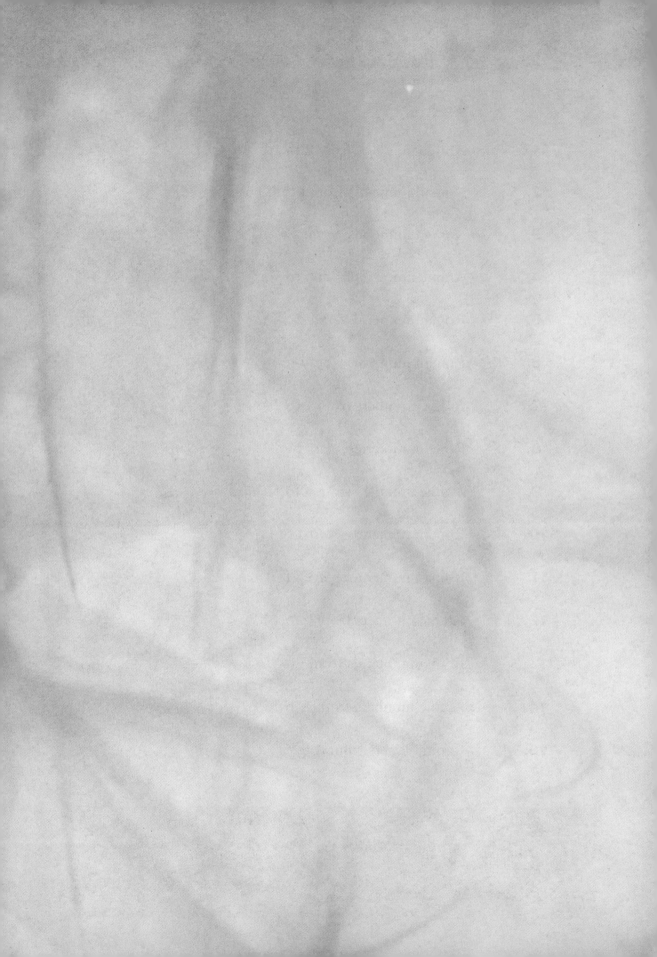

English Language and Composition

Basic Grammar
Rules and Exceptions

BOS Statement

Correct the originator's obvious grammatical errors.

Where?
BOS p. 196

Grammar refers to the set of rules governing a particular language. It is part of the overall study of language known as *linguistics*. Every language, whether formal or dialectical, has its own grammar—rules that govern the whys and hows of that language. While it may seem that grammar is only learned by formal instruction, the truth is that all languages have an inherent grammar that can be observed in a child long before that child enters "grammar school." Languages that arise in regions of blended ethnicity, for example, will naturally develop not only content but also a consistent pattern of grammar. For that reason, linguists often refer to *prescriptive* and *descriptive* grammars. Prescriptive grammars are those used by prestige groups within a language community, those that condemn the use of certain constructions that fall outside mainstream acceptability. Descriptive grammars represent the language that is actually used by people (e.g., the use of "ain't" or double negatives in speech). Modern linguists prefer descriptive grammar because it more accurately represents the way language is spoken and not the way a certain group or influence perceives that it *should* be spoken.

The business community, however, follows suit with the academic community in subscribing to prescriptive grammar in the English language in order to ensure consistency, standards, and clear communication. Healthcare documentation is no exception. The standard of expectation is that these records will reflect both accuracy and *quality*, the latter of which speaks to the grammatically correct expression of the healthcare information being outlined. It will be your responsibility as a medical transcriptionist to ensure that the record reflects that standard.

Going Deeper

Strong language skills are critical to the skilled MT, and they will often make the difference between an average transcriptionist and an excellent one. An understanding of language structure and the rules related to sentence construction and agreement, for example, will be essential to identifying grammatical errors in dictation and correcting them in the transcribed record.

It is the reality of the profession that you will encounter variable language skills among the dictators for whom you will provide transcription. Many dictators have poor fundamental grammar themselves; others speak English as a second language and possess only a rudimentary grasp of the language. Still others will be careless or hurried and will make errors that you will be expected to recognize and correct. In other words, you will not be able to simply rely on the skills of the dictator. If the physician dictates, "Lungs is clear," you will be expected to correct it.

If you do not have a good grasp of language and grammar, now would be a good time to invest in a comprehensive language text (such as *The Gregg Reference Manual*) for more in-depth study. The sections of *The AAMT Book of Style* that refer to grammar standards provide a general overview only and assume that the MT will have covered this information in more depth either prior to, during, or beyond the classroom. You may have forgotten the fundamental grammar concepts you learned in school and may need a refresher course in parts of speech, sentence construction, subject/verb agreement, and diction beyond what is covered below.

Rules & Exceptions

Parts of Speech

adjectives

Adjectives modify nouns and sometimes pronouns.

Use commas to separate two or more adjectives if each modifies the noun alone. Do not place a comma between the last adjective and the modified noun.

> **Physical exam reveals a pleasant, cooperative, slender lady in no acute distress.**
> **The abdomen is soft, nontender, and supple.**

However, do not place a comma after an adjective that modifies a combination of the adjective(s) and noun that follow it.

> **This 54-year-old Caucasian female was referred to my office for evaluation.**
> **She did not have audible paroxysmal tachycardia.**

Use commas to set off an adjective or adjectival phrase directly following the noun it modifies.

> DIAGNOSIS
>
> **Fracture, left tibia.**
> **He has degenerative arthritis, left knee, with increasing inability to cope.**
> **Blood cultures, all of which were negative, were drawn at 4-hour intervals.**

Some words can function as adjectives or adverbs, depending on how they are used.

adjective	adverb
hard work	play *hard*
light color	travel *light*

HINT: If you can replace the comma between adjectives with *and*, the comma is necessary.

adverbs

Adverbs modify verbs, adjectives, and other adverbs. Some but not all adverbs end in -ly.

sterilely

An adverb may be placed between the parts of a compound verb, provided it does not obstruct the meaning.

He will routinely return for followup.

It is increasingly acceptable to split an infinitive verb (e.g., the verb *to be*) with an adverb. Transcribe as dictated, provided the phrasing does not obstruct the meaning.

The test was expected to definitively determine the diagnosis.

squinting modifiers

A squinting modifier is an adverb that is placed in such a way that it can be interpreted as modifying more than one word. If the intended meaning can be determined, recast the sentence so that the modifier clearly relates to the appropriate word. See how the placement of *only* in the following sentence changes the meaning.

He only walked 2 blocks. *(He only walked, not ran.)*
Only he walked 2 blocks. *(Only he, not anyone else, walked 2 blocks.)*
He walked only 2 blocks. *(He didn't walk more than 2 blocks.)*

So the squinting modifier *only* in "He only walked 2 blocks" should be moved so that the sentence reads "He walked only 2 blocks."

articles

Articles (*a, an, the*) are modifiers that are used to indicate the definiteness (*the*) or indefiniteness (*a, an*) of the noun that follows. Articles are frequently dropped in dictation. They may be transcribed or not (whether dictated or not) provided their presence or absence does not substantially change the meaning or style of the originator. Articles are more apt to be included in correspondence than in reports. When dropped in transcription, it is usually because they were not dictated, they were not heard by the transcriptionist, or they were not dictated elsewhere in the report and the transcriptionist is attempting to achieve some consistency within the document.

The use of articles with abbreviations varies. Sometimes the article is required. Sometimes it is optional. Sometimes it should be omitted.

Required:	**We will do a CBC.**
Optional:	**She was admitted to the ICU.**
	or
	She was admitted to ICU.
Omission required:	**CPR was done . . .**
	not
	The CPR was done . . .

conjunctions

Words that join words, phrases, or clauses, thereby indicating their relationship. Examples: *and, but, for, however, or, nor, yet, so.*

conjunctive adverbs

Conjunctive adverbs connect two independent clauses. They include *consequently, finally, furthermore, however, moreover, nevertheless, similarly, subsequently, then, therefore, thus.* Precede a conjunctive adverb by a semicolon (sometimes a period), and usually follow it by a comma.

> She reported feeling better; however, her fever still spiked in the evenings.
> He was admitted through the emergency room; then he was taken to surgery.

coordinating conjunctions

Coordinating conjunctions (*and, but, or, nor, for*) join separate main clauses. They are usually preceded by a comma, sometimes by a semicolon, occasionally a colon.

> He was seen in the emergency room, but he was not admitted.

Do not use a comma before a coordinating conjunction that is followed by a second verb without a new subject.

> The patient tolerated the procedure well and left the department in stable condition.
> The gallbladder was inflamed but without stones.

subordinating conjunctions

Subordinating conjunctions (*while, where, since, after, yet, so*) connect two unequal parts, e.g., dependent and independent clauses. Precede a subordinating conjunction by a comma in most cases.

> He was in great pain, yet he refused treatment.

correlative conjunctions

Terms or phrases used in pairs, e.g., *either . . . or, neither . . . nor,* and *not only . . . but also*.

With an *either . . . or* or *neither . . . nor* construction, match the number of the verb with the number of the nearest subject.

> Neither the sister nor the brothers exhibit similar symptoms.
> Neither the brothers nor the sister exhibits similar symptoms.

If the subjects before and after *or* or *nor* are both singular, use a singular verb; if both subjects are plural, use a plural verb.

> **Neither the sister nor the brother exhibits similar symptoms.**
> **Neither the sisters nor the brothers exhibit similar symptoms.**

With *not only . . . but also*, check usage for parallelism; recast as necessary. If *also* is omitted, insert it or some other word(s) for balance.

> DICTATED
> **He could not only be stubborn but offensive.**
>
> TRANSCRIBED
> **He could be not only stubborn but also offensive.**
>
> *or*
>
> **He could be not only stubborn but offensive as well.**

nouns

Proper nouns name specific persons, places, and things. All other nouns are common nouns. It may help to think of proper nouns as brand names and common nouns as generic terms. Do not capitalize common nouns in an attempt to give them the stature of proper nouns.

> **He was admitted to *St. Mary's Hospital. (proper noun)***
> **She was seen in the *emergency room* of St. Mary's Hospital. *(common noun)***

Nouns usually are subjects or objects of a sentence. Sometimes, they may be modifiers.

> **She became ill while attending an *educators* conference. (*not* educators' conference)**

Use the possessive form for a noun or pronoun that precedes a gerund (verb ending in *-ing* and used as a noun).

> His *dieting* is a problem.
> The *patient's screaming* disturbed other patients.

Use the possessive form for a noun involving time, measurement, or money that is used as a possessive adjective.

> The pain was of 3 months' duration.

collective noun

Represents a collection of persons or things regarded as a unit. Usage determines whether the collective noun is singular or plural. It is singular and takes a singular verb when the total group it represents is emphasized. It is plural and takes a plural verb when the individuals making up the group are emphasized. Examples of collective nouns: *board (of directors), majority, class, number, committee, pair, couple, set, family, staff, group,* and *team.*

> The group is meeting frequently throughout its stay.
> The group of patients were female. *(each was female)*
> A number of adhesions were present. *(individual adhesions were present, not a collective adhesion)*
> The number of adhesions was minimal. *(The subject* the number of *always takes a singular verb.)*
> The couple were injured in a plane crash.
>
> *but*
>
> The couple has an appointment with the geneticist.

Treat units of measure as singular collective nouns that take singular verbs.

> **At 8:30 this morning, 20 mEq of KCl was administered.**

prepositions　A preposition relates to its object, either a noun or a pronoun.

> **The patient was taken into the delivery room. (*Into* is the preposition; *delivery room* is its object.)**

Pronouns following prepositions must be in the objective case: *me, us, it, you, him, her, them.*

> **between you and me**
> **not between you and I**

The following is a list of common prepositions: *about, across, after, against, along, among, around, at, before, below, beneath, beside, between, by, down, during, except, for, from, in, inside, into, like, near, of, off, on, outside, over, past, through, to, toward, under, underneath, until, up, with, within,* and *without.*

pronouns – personal　Personal pronouns have person and number as well as subjective (S), possessive (P), and objective (O) forms.

	S	P	O
first person singular	I	mine	me
first person plural	we	ours	us
second person singular	you	yours	you
second person plural	you	yours	you
third person singular	he/she/it	his/hers/its	him/her/it
third person plural	they	theirs	them

The personal pronoun must agree in number and gender with the preceding noun or pronoun to which it refers.

> **The patient was sent to the postpartum floor. She improved steadily.**

Do not use an apostrophe with possessive pronouns. In particular, be careful not to confuse *its* with *it's*. *Its* (no apostrophe) is the possessive form of *it*. *It's* is the contraction form of *it is* or *it has*.

> **my conclusion**
> **your referral**
> **his review of systems**
> **our plan**
> **its significance (*not* it's)**
> **ours *not* our's**
> **theirs *not* their's**
> **yours *not* your's**

pronouns – reflexive

Reflexive pronouns are pronouns combined with *-self* or *-selves*. They refer to and emphasize the subject of the verb.

> **She insisted on feeding herself.**

Avoid other uses of reflexive pronouns.

> DICTATED
> **The patient will be seen by Dr. Smith in 1 week and by myself in 2 weeks.**
>
> TRANSCRIBED
> **The patient will be seen by Dr. Smith in 1 week and by me in 2 weeks.**

pronouns – relative

Relative pronouns (*that, who, whom, what, which*, and their variations *whoever, whomever, whosoever, whatever, whichever*) refer to previous nouns as they introduce subordinate clauses.

Use *who* or *whom* to introduce an **essential** clause referring to a human being or to an animal with a name.

Use *that* to introduce an **essential** clause referring to an inanimate object or to an animal without a name. Exception: When *that* as a conjunction is used elsewhere in the same sentence, use *which*, not *that*, to introduce an essential clause.

Do not use commas to set off **essential** subordinate clauses.

> **The patient came into the emergency room, and she was treated for tachycardia that had resisted conversion in her physician's office.**
> **He had 2 large wounds that were bleeding profusely and several small bleeders.**
> **She said that the dog which bit her was a miniature poodle.**

Use *who* or *whom* to introduce a **nonessential** clause referring to a human being or to an animal with a name.

Use *which* to introduce a **nonessential** clause referring to an inanimate object or to an animal without a name.

Precede and follow a **nonessential** clause with a comma or closing punctuation.

> **The surgery, which had been postponed 3 times, was finally performed today.**
> **The patient's parents, who had been summoned from Europe, were consulted about her past history.**

pronouns without antecedents

Text with a pronoun that does not have a preceding noun or pronoun should be edited to identify the pronoun's antecedent.

> DICTATED
> **She is a 40-year-old white female complaining of nausea and vomiting. *(first sentence of report)***
>
> TRANSCRIBED
> **The patient is a 40-year-old white female complaining of nausea and vomiting.**

verbs

Verbs express action or being. Verbs have mood, person and number, tense, and voice.

The *indicative* mood makes factual statements and is most common.

> **The patient returned on schedule for a followup visit.**

The *imperative* mood makes requests or demands.

> **Come here now.**

The *subjunctive* mood expresses doubt, wishes, regrets, or conditions contrary to fact. It is the most difficult and most formal mood and usually relates to the past or present, not the future.

indicative	**He is a singer.**
imperative	**Clean up your room.**
subjunctive	**If she were my patient, I would proceed with surgery.**

Person expresses the entity (first, second, or third) that is acting or being. *Number* expresses whether the person is singular or plural.

first person singular	**I**
second person	**singular you** *(one only)*
third person singular	**he, she,** *or* **it**
first person plural	**we**
second person plural	**you** *(more than one)*
third person plural	**they**

Use verb tense to communicate the appropriate time of the action or being: past, present, future, past perfect, present perfect, and future perfect. Maintain uniformity of tense, but keep in mind that tense may vary within a single report or even a single paragraph, depending on the time being referenced.

> DICTATED
> **The abdomen is soft. There was a scar in the lower right quadrant.**
>
> TRANSCRIBED
> **The abdomen is soft. There is a scar in the lower right quadrant.**

Tenses may appropriately vary within a single paragraph and certainly within a report.

> **She was admitted from the emergency room at 8:30 p.m. She is afebrile at present. She will be given IV antibiotics, nevertheless.**

The *historic present tense* uses the present tense to relate past events in a more immediate manner. In dictation, it is common to use the historic present tense to describe patient information or treatment in the present rather than in the past. If this is done, be consistent. The historic present is not the same as the universal present.

> **The *patient says she has* pain over the right abdomen.**
> **Upon examination, *there is* rebound tenderness.**

The *universal present tense* uses the present tense to state something that is universally true or that was believed to be true at the time. The universal present is not the same as the historic present.

> **Traditional treatment modalities were used because *they are* so effective.**

In the *active voice*, the subject is the doer. In the *passive voice*, the subject is done unto. Most communication guidelines urge use of the active voice except when it is more important to emphasize **what** was acted on and that it **was** acted on.

In medical transcription, the active voice is more common in reporting observations, e.g., in history and physical exam reports, while the passive voice is more common in describing healthcare providers' actions, e.g., hospital treatment and surgery.

> **The abdomen is soft, nontender.**
> **The patient was given intravenous aminophylline.**
> **The incision was made over the symphysis pubis.**

Do not recast most dictation to change the voice except for those sentences that are especially awkward.

> DICTATED
> **The medication by him is taken irregularly.**
>
> TRANSCRIBED
> **He takes the medication irregularly.**

linking verbs   Verbs that link the subject of a sentence to an adjective or other complement. Most common examples are various forms of the verb *to be*. Others include *act, appear, feel, look, remain, become, get, grow, seem, smell, sound,* and *taste.*

Such verbs are followed by adjectives, not adverbs, because the subject, not the verb, is being described.

> **He says the food tastes bad.**
>
> *not*
>
> **He says the food tastes badly.**

split verbs   A split verb is one in which a word (usually an adverb) has been inserted between its two parts. Splitting infinitives or other forms of verbs used to be considered a grave grammatical faux pas. Traditionalists still hold to this view, but pragmatists recognize that such splits are appropriate if they enhance meaning (or at least do not obstruct it).

Transcribe split verbs as dictated provided they do not obstruct the meaning.

10.4

> The test was intended *to* definitively *determine*.
> He *will* routinely *return* for followup.

unnecessary verbs

In comparisons such as the following, the second verb is understood.

> The larger incision healed faster than the smaller one.

If the second verb is dictated or added, be sure to place it at the end.

> The larger incision healed faster than the smaller one did.
>
> *not*
>
> The larger incision healed faster than did the smaller one.

SUBJECT-VERB AGREEMENT

subject-verb agreement

A verb must agree in number and person with the noun that serves as its subject. Use a singular verb with a singular subject, a plural verb with a plural subject.

> The abdomen is soft and nontender.
> The lungs are clear.

Exception: *You* always takes a plural verb.

> You are late for your appointment.

The verb must agree with its subject even when the two are not in proximity. Be especially careful when another noun intervenes.

> The *findings* on tomography *were* normal.
> (The subject is *findings*, not *tomography*.)
> The products of conception were examined.
> (The subject is *products*, not *conception*.)
> What surprised me was that the symptoms were not typical.
> (The subject of the sentence is *what surprised me*, not *the symptoms*, which is the subject of the dependent clause, so the verb is singular.)

HINT: A phrase or clause acting as a subject requires a singular verb.

compound subjects

Compound subjects joined by *and* always take a plural verb, except when both subjects refer to the same person or thing.

> **The date and time of the accident are not certain.**
>
> *but*
>
> **Spaghetti and meatballs was our first course.**

Compound subjects joined by *or* or *nor* may take a singular or plural verb, depending on the subject situated closest to the verb in the sentence.

> **Neither the kidneys nor the spleen was palpated.**
>
> *but*
>
> **Neither the spleen nor the kidneys were palpated.**

collective nouns

Collective nouns may be singular or plural, and they take the matching verb.

> **The family is in agreement on the patient's care.**
> *(emphasizes the family as a unit)*
>
> *or*
>
> **The family are in agreement on the patient's care.**
> *(emphasizes the individual members of the family)*

time, money, and quantity

When referring to a total amount, use a singular verb. When referring to a number of individual units, use a plural verb.

> **Three weeks is a long time.**
> **Five days have passed.**
> **In all, 4 doses were given, and 20 mEq was given this morning.**

pronouns

If the subject is a pronoun, be careful to determine what the pronoun is referring to.

> **He is one of those patients who demand constant reassurance.**
> **(The subject of *demand* is *who*, referring to *patients*, not *he*.)**

irregular nouns

Some nouns always take a singular verb.

> **The ascites was tapped for the third time.**
> **The patient's lues has progressed over many years' time.**

Some nouns always take a plural verb.

> **The left uterine adnexa were entirely involved with tumor.**
> **The right ocular adnexa are within normal limits.**

Some nouns retain the same form, whether singular or plural.

> The left biceps was weaker than the right.
> The left and right biceps were equally strong.
> A scissors was used to cut . . .
> An Allis forceps was used to grasp . . .
> Several different-sized scissors were used.
> Both forceps were required to grasp . . .
> A series of tests was conducted.
> Several series of tests were conducted.

units of measure

Units of measure are collective singular nouns and take singular verbs.

> After the lab report came back, 20 mEq of KCl was added.
> 3 mL was injected

The Final Word

While grammar is rarely a critical concern in healthcare documentation from a clinical accuracy perspective, few could argue its important role in creating a credible document. A thorough understanding of English language and the application of grammar represent the kind of "polish" that an MT is expected to bring to the documentation process. Providers are often most concerned with making sure they dictate all of the pertinent clinical information. Those that are in a hurry to document and those that speak English as a second language may be challenged to dictate in an organized, logical way that facilitates precise grammar. The MT transcribing for those providers will need to be on his/her proverbial toes, translating those hurried clips of clinical information into a clean, credible care record.

Test Your Knowledge

I. The following paragraph contains numbered *italicized* words. For each, indicate the part of speech (*noun, verb, adjective, adverb, pronoun, preposition, or conjunction*). For the *nouns, verbs, pronouns* and *conjunctions*, indicate the type.

The (1) *patient* presented to the office (2) *with* a complaint of (3) *shortness* of breath (4) *and* productive cough (5) *although* it (6) *has* been of (7) *short* duration. On (8) *my* evaluation (9) *today*, she appeared (10) *tired* and ill. (11) *Her* skin was (12) *slightly* dry, indicating (13) *some* dehydration. There was some (14) *redness* of the throat, and her nose showed moist (15) *but* congested (16) *mucous* membranes. (17) *When* I auscultated (18) *the* lungs, they were clear (19) *bilaterally*, and breath sounds were equal on (20) *both* sides.

II. For each of the following sentences, <u>underline</u> the subject of the sentence and circle the verb that agrees with that subject.

1. The cause of heartbeats (*has, have*) been a subject of continuous inquiry in the scientific community.

2. The heartbeat, as well as other factors, (*cause, causes*) blood to flow throughout the body.

3. H. Allen and others (*has, have*) shown that the control of the nervous system is not linked to the beating of the heart.

4. The power of contractions (*belong, belongs*) to the cardiac muscle itself, unassisted by other impulses.

5.   Each of the strips of muscle in the heart (*is, are*) capable of rhythmic action.

6.   The power to trigger contractions (*differ, differs*) throughout the heart.

7.   Every one of these contractions (*originate, originates*) from the centralization of greatest energy at the top of the heart.

8.   The lesser energies of the heart (*is, are*) centered toward the bottom.

9.   The number of beats of the heart per minute usually (*decline, declines*) with age, from as much as 140 at birth to 50 in an adult male.

10.   The sequence of events in a single heartbeat (*is, are*) complex and worth studying.

Test Your Knowledge

Answers

I.

1.	noun
2.	preposition
3.	noun
4.	conjunction (coordinating)
5.	conjunction (subordinating)
6.	verb (linking)
7.	adjective
8.	pronoun (possessive) *Note: "adjective" also acceptable answer.*
9.	adverb
10.	adjective
11.	pronoun (possessive) *Note: "adjective" also acceptable answer.*
12.	adverb
13.	adjective
14.	noun

15. conjunction (coordinating)

16. adjective

17. conjunction (subordinating)

18. adjective

19. adverb

20. adjective

II.

1. has

2. causes

3. have

4. belongs

5. is

6. differs

7. originates

8. are

9. declines

10. is

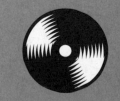

APPLICATION TEST
Take the application test for this chapter on your CD-ROM.
Access the section for
Chapter 10: "Basic Grammar."

Capitalization

BOS Statement

Where?
BOS pp. 56–57

Capitals emphasize and draw attention to the terms in which they are used. Use them appropriately and judiciously because their overuse diminishes their value and impact.

Some words are always capitalized, some never. The placement or use of a term may determine whether it is capitalized. Capitals, for example, are always used to mark the beginning of a sentence.

Learning and adopting the rules of capitalization, when they should be used and when they should not be used, as well as the few instances when variations may be acceptable, will improve the consistency, accuracy, and communication value of transcribed healthcare documents.

In particular, avoid the use of unnecessary or inappropriate capitals. Do not, for example, capitalize a common-noun reference to a thing or person if it is just one of many other such things or persons. Thus, *emergency room and recovery room* are not capitalized. Think of the rule for generic versus brand names for drugs. The generic term (common noun) *emergency room* is applied to all emergency rooms, so it is not capitalized.

Going Deeper

Capital letters serve many purposes. They serve to indicate the beginning of sentences and are an integral aid to the reader. They distinguish names, titles and proper nouns from the rest of the sentence. Some, however, are merely conventions. They are usages adopted by people of formal education for no other reason than that they are customary. Conventional usage of capitalization sets the standard of expectation in formal writing.

As in all other areas of language usage, inconsistencies can be found in the application of rules related to capitalization. In standard usage, for example, the names of seasons are not capitalized, but many print publications choose to capitalize them. Many of the rules outlined below will caution you to verify that the entity in question customarily capitalizes any or all of the words that refer to that entity. For example, it is important to know that "3M" is trademarked that way, with the Arabic numeral and capital M without a space in between. This is where knowledge about proper names and/or the ability to verify them will be essential.

Nowhere do we see this dilemma more consistently in transcription than with drug names. As you will note below, and remember from Chapter 8, medical transcriptionists are expected to recognize when a dictated medication is either brand or generic and capitalize only brand-name medications. This means that as an MT, you will not be able to apply a blanket rule for capitalization in these critical areas of the report. Good referencing skills and a sound memorization of the most common drugs over time will ultimately serve you best.

Rules & Exceptions

Capitalization

academic degrees

Do not capitalize generic forms of academic degrees.

> **bachelor's degree**
> **master's**

Capitalize the expanded form only when it follows a person's name.

> **Jane Smith, Licensed Clinical Social Worker**

acronyms

Capitalize all letters of most acronyms, but when they are extended, do not capitalize the words from which they are formed unless they are proper names.

> **AIDS (acquired immunodeficiency syndrome)**
> **BiPAP (bilateral positive airway pressure)**
> **TURP (transurethral resection of prostate)**

When acronyms become words in their own right, they sometimes evolve into lowercase form. Many users of these terms are not aware that such terms are acronyms and do not know what terms the letters represent.

> **laser (light amplification by stimulated emission of radiation)**
> **scuba (self-contained underwater breathing apparatus)**

Check appropriate references (dictionaries, abbreviation books) to determine current preferred forms and usage.

assistant/ associate

Do not capitalize unless used in a formal address or when part of a formal title before a name, such as in a signature line. Examples of capitalization of assistant and associate in text are rare because the terms usually represent job or occupational titles, not formal titles (even when placed before a name). Do not abbreviate.

Set off with commas if the title is descriptive without the name or if the title is used to further identify the person.

> **The assistant surgeon, Dr. Jones, closed the wound.**
>
> *or*
>
> **Dr. Jones, assistant surgeon, closed the wound.**

Capitalize when used in a formal address or signature line.

> **Richard Jones, MD**
> **Associate Professor of Clinical Psychiatry**

business names

Express according to the business's style and usage. Use the full name before using the abbreviated form in order to avoid confusion among similar abbreviations except for businesses, such as IBM, that are better known by their abbreviations than by their full names.

In general, use initial caps for all words in a business name except articles and prepositions or words that the business chooses to lowercase.

> **eBay**

Capitalize words such as *organization, institution, association* only when they are part of the entity's official name; do not capitalize them when they are used alone or in a shortened version of the name. Note: The entity, in shortened references to itself, may choose to use initial capitals.

> **American Hospital Association**
>
> *but*
>
> **the association**
>
> *or*
>
> **the hospital association**

company, Company

Capitalize *company* only if part of an official name.

> **Campbell Soup Company**
> **company policy**

Co., Corp., Inc., Ltd.

Abbreviate and capitalize *Co.*, *Corp.*, *Inc.*, or *Ltd.* only when the business being named uses the abbreviation in its formal name. Do not use a comma before *Inc.* or *Ltd.* unless the specific entity uses it.

> **Ford Motor Co.**

credentials, professional

Capitalize abbreviated forms, but do not capitalize the extended form unless it follows a person's name.

> **a CMT**
> **a certified medical transcriptionist**
> **James Morrison, CMT**
> **Jane Smith, Doctor of Medicine**

departments

Lowercase common nouns designating department names; reserve capitals for proper nouns or adjectives, in addresses, or when part of a federal government agency name.

> **She is head of the St. Mary's Hospital surgery department.**
> **He works for the State Department in Washington, DC.**
> **The patient is head of the English department at the local state university.**

However, capitalize a department name that is referred to as an entity.

> **The patient was referred to Anesthesia for pre-operative evaluation.**
> **The report from Pathology indicates that the tumor is benign.**

divisions

Lowercase common nouns naming institutional divisions.

> **the administrative division of Memorial Hospital**

199

internal units   Lowercase common names for internal units of an organization.

> **The patient's medication was changed because apparently the pharmacy can no longer obtain paregoric.**

Exception: Capitalization may be used for such internal units in the entity's references to itself in its own formal and/or legal documents.

> **Please note the change in Pharmacy hours...**

Capitalize internal elements when their names are not generic terms.

> **Dr. Smith's Limb Deficiency Clinic**

inverted forms   When inverted forms of names are widely used and recognized, capitalize those forms as well.

> **College of William and Mary**
> **William and Mary College**

drug terminology   **Brand names.** The brand name is the manufacturer's name for a drug; it is the same as the trade name, trademark, or proprietary name. It may suggest a use or indication, and it often incorporates the manufacturer's name.

Capitalize brand names, trade names, and trademark names.

> **Tagamet**
> **Bayer**

Use of idiosyncratic capitalization is optional.

> **pHisoHex**
>
> *or*
>
> **Phisohex**

The trade name is a broader term than trademark, identifying the manufacturer but not the product.

Capitalize trade names.

> **Dr. Scholl's**

Generic names. The generic name is also known as the nonproprietary name, the established, official name for a drug. In the United States, it is created by the US Adopted Names Council (USAN). International nomenclature is coordinated by the World Health Organization. Generic names are in the public domain; their use is unrestricted.

Do not capitalize generic names. When the generic name and brand name of a medication sound alike, use the generic spelling unless it is certain that the brand name is being referenced.

> **aminophylline (generic name)**
>
> *not*
>
> **Aminophyllin (brand name)**

eponyms　　Capitalize eponyms but not the common nouns, adjectives, and prefixes that accompany them.

> **Homans sign**
> **Lyme disease**
> **Down syndrome**

Do not capitalize words derived from eponyms.

> **ligament of Treitz**
> **red Robinson catheter**
> **non-Hodgkin lymphoma**
> **Parkinson disease** *but* **parkinsonism**
> **Cushing syndrome** *but* **cushingoid**

genus and species names

Always capitalize genus names and their abbreviated forms when they are accompanied by a species name.

Always lowercase species names.

> **Haemophilus influenzae**
> **Escherichia coli**
> **Staphylococcus aureus**

Lowercase genus names used in plural and adjectival forms and when used in the vernacular, for example, when they stand alone (without a species name).

> **staphylococcus**
> **group B streptococcus**
> **staphylococci**
> **staphylococcal infection**
> **staph infection**
> **strep throat**

The suffixes *-osis* and *-iasis* indicate disease caused by a particular class of infectious agents or types of infection. Lowercase terms formed with these suffixes.

> **amebiasis**
> **dermatophytosis**

geographic names

Capitalize names of political divisions such as streets, cities, towns, counties, states, countries; topographic names, e.g., mountains, rivers, oceans, islands; and accepted designations for regions.

> **the Bay Area**
> **Great Britain**
> **Lake Wobegon**
> **the Middle East**
> **Wallingford Avenue**
> **Yosemite National Park**

Capitalize common nouns that are an official part of a proper name; lowercase them when they stand alone.

> **Philippine Islands**
> **the islands**

Capitalize compass directions when they are part of the geographic name.

> **East Timor**

Capitalize geographic names used as eponyms.

> **Lyme disease**

Do not capitalize words derived from geographic names when they have a special meaning.

> **india ink**
> **plaster of paris**
> **french fries**

parenthetical expressions If the parenthetical entry is within a sentence, begin it with a lowercase letter and omit closing punctuation whether or not it is a complete sentence.

> **Further past history shows outpatient pulmonary function tests with a forced vital capacity of 2.57 liters (equal to 62% of predicted) and an FEV1 of 0.98 liters.**

A parenthetical entry that stands on its own (is not simply a part of a sentence) must be a complete sentence;

start it with a capital letter and end it with closing punctuation inside the closing parenthesis.

> **Pelvic ultrasound was read as intrauterine changes consistent with pyometra. (It is difficult to believe that this diagnosis could be made on the basis of an ultrasound.)**

personal names

Capitalize personal names.

> **Stanley Livingston**

For foreign names, follow the person's preference for spelling, spacing and capitalization. Capitalize or lowercase the foreign particles *de, du, di, d', le, la, l', van, von, ter,* etc., according to the preference of the individual named. Check appropriate references for guidance. Use lowercase if unable to determine preference. When a lowercase particle begins a sentence, it must be capitalized.

> **De Pezzer catheters were used.**
>
> *but*
>
> **We inserted a de Pezzer catheter.**
> **a DeBakey procedure**

personifications

Capitalize personifications, such as Mother Nature.

> **He kept saying, "You can't fool Mother Nature."**
> **We called Pathology and they reported a negative reading on the specimen.**

quotations

Begin a complete quotation with a capital letter if it is not grammatically joined to what precedes it.

> **Path report reads, "Specimen is consistent with microadenoma."**

Do not use a capital letter to begin incomplete quotations or those joined grammatically to what precedes them.

> **She says that she has "bad blood."**

Capitalize the first word in a direct question even if the question is not placed within quotation marks.

> **She refused to answer the question, What is your name?**

NOTE: Be careful not to include language within the quotation that is not a direct quote, despite what may be dictated. Recast the sentence to include only a direct quote within the quotation marks.

> DICTATED
> **The patient says quote her back hurts unquote.**
>
> TRANSCRIBED
> **The patient says her "back hurts."**
>
> *or*
>
> **The patient says, "My back hurts."**
>
> *not*
>
> **The patient says "her back hurts."**

sociocultural designations

Capitalize the names of languages, peoples, races, religions, political parties.

> **Caucasian**
> **Chinese**
> **Filipino**
> **Methodist**
> **Republican**

Color designations of race and ethnicity are usually not capitalized. However, some publications capitalize Black to identify African Americans.

> **75-year-old black woman**
> **85-year-old white man**

Sexual preferences or orientations are not capitalized.

> **gay**
> **heterosexual**
> **lesbian**

state, county, city & town

Always capitalize the initial letter of a state, county, city, or town name or a resident designation.

> **Boston, Massachusetts**
> **Bostonian**

Lowercase the phrase *county of* unless referring to a county's government.

Lowercase generic uses, including use as an adjective to refer to a level of government.

> **The county of Stanislaus includes Modesto, California.**
> **The County of Stanislaus held a budget hearing.**
> **Assessment of county highways . . .**

Lowercase the phrase *state of* unless referring to a state's government.

Lowercase generic uses, including use as an adjective to refer to a level of government.

> **The state of California has many geographies.**
> **The State of California challenged the federal mandate.**
> **state coffers**
> **state highways**

Lowercase the phrase *city of* unless referring to a city's government. Lowercase generic uses, including use as an adjective to refer to a level of government. The same guidelines apply to *town, village,* etc.

> **The city of Modesto is growing steadily.**
> **The City of Modesto challenged the state mandate.**

Capitalize *city* or similar term only if an integral part of an official name or commonly used name or nickname, or in official references. Otherwise, lowercase. The same guidelines apply to *town, village,* etc.

> **New York City**
> **City of Commerce (official name of city)**
> **the Windy City**
> **The town budget was reviewed.**

In titles, capitalize *city* or similar term only if part of a formal title placed before a name; lowercase when not part of a formal title or when the title follows the name. The same guidelines apply to *town, village,* etc.

> **City Manager Dixon**
> **William Howard, city supervisor**

The Final Word

The fundamental role of capitalization is to give distinction, importance, or emphasis to words. A word is capitalized at the beginning of a sentence, for example, to clearly delineate that a new sentence has begun. In that role, capital letters serve as visual markers that assist the reader in transitioning from one concept to the next. Most words, however, are capitalized primarily to emphasize their identities as entities of significance. The medical transcriptionist who is expected to recognize those myriad entities will need to be knowledgeable and possess excellent referencing skills in order to ensure their accurate inclusion. Some terms (like *board of directors*) may function either as proper nouns or as common nouns, and an interpretive eye that understands the significance of those terms *in context* will be necessary in determining their application. Given the debate over the use of capitalization in formal writing (some experts feel that overusing capitalization results in the reality that when too many words stand out, *none* stand out), it is always important to let the need for clarity guide you in the use of capitalization for emphasis.

Test Your Knowledge

Each of the sentences below contains at least one error in capitalization. Correct each error.

1. The patient was combative on examination, kicking and yelling "leave me alone" when I tried to evaluate her.

2. She was transferred to the Postsurgical Care Unit.

3. He was diagnosed with Rocky Mountain Spotted Fever in his early 20s.

4. She admits to smoking a pack and a half a day (She has apparently tried to quit twice.) and drinks occasionally.

5. She saw Dr. Clark originally for her Von Willebrand disease, but she is presently under Dr. Smith's management for this.

6. Her culture grew out group-B Streptococcus.

7. This is a 32-year-old White male in no acute distress.

8. He has worked for the city of Jacksonville for 13 years.

9. She was given rhogam after her first pregnancy.

10. Does this say "take twice a day?"

Test Your Knowledge

Answers

1. The patient was combative on examination, kicking and yelling, "Leave me alone!" when I tried to evaluate her.

2. She was transferred to the postsurgical care unit.

3. He was diagnosed with Rocky Mountain spotted fever in his early 20s.

4. She admits to smoking a pack and a half a day (she has apparently tried to quit twice) and drinks occasionally.

5. She saw Dr. Clark originally for her von Willebrand disease, but she is presently under Dr. Smith's management for this.

6. Her culture grew out group-B streptococcus.

7. This is a 32-year-old white male in no acute distress.

8. He has worked for the City of Jacksonville for 13 years.

9. She was given Rhogam after her first pregnancy.
   or
   She was given RhoGAM after her first pregnancy.

10. Does this say, "Take twice a day"?

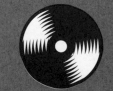

APPLICATION TEST
Take the application test for this chapter on your CD-ROM.
Access the section for
Chapter 11: "Capitalization."

Punctuation

BOS Statement

Follow punctuation rules and use punctuation to enhance the clarity and accuracy of the communication. Do not make exceptions without being able to justify doing so. Omit punctuation not required by punctuation rules and not needed for clarity and/or accuracy. Consult specific entries in this book and other appropriate references (e.g., grammar book) for guidance.

Where?
BOS p. 340

Going Deeper

Punctuation marks serve a vital role in sentence construction. They are relationship indicators when word order alone is not sufficient to convey meaning. Without major punctuation, there would be no visual boundaries around the written word to guide the reader from one concept, or idea, to the next. Without punctuation, documentation would be a visual mess.

As a medical transcriptionist, you will be tasked with accurately punctuating the sentences dictated to you; the knack of incorporating this into the natural flow of your transcription will develop over time. This area of transcription can be particularly frustrating to the MT, since physicians do not always dictate sentence flow in a manner that facilitates clean punctuation, and many will attempt to dictate punctuation where it should not be placed.

This is one of the few areas in the report where MTs are encouraged *not* to rely on physician direction. As with spelling, physicians cannot always be relied upon to provide accurate direction with punctuation. Many will attempt to dictate punctuation as part of the report. Occasionally, you will encounter a dictator who possesses the language skills that might make this helpful. However, this is not always the case. A physician whose primary skill set lies in the clinical arena cannot be relied upon to have advanced writing skills, and it is the MT's responsibility to ensure that punctuation is judiciously applied to the patient record.

Knowledge of punctuation rules and a very clear understanding of applying these rules will be essential to producing a quality document. An MT who is relying on a vague or "general" understanding of punctuation will encounter difficulty in this area. For example, some people are under the mistaken impression that commas should be placed anywhere that you "pause" in the sentence. An MT will quickly discover that this rule is impossible to apply to dictation that is delivered by providers who either chronically pause throughout their dictation or *never* pause from the moment they begin a report until they sign off from it.

There are many clear rules governing the placement of punctuation in formal writing. MTs should avoid the random and haphazard placement of punctuation, particularly commas, and begin to develop a substantive ability to analyze sentences; determine the role and function of the words, phrases, and clauses within those sentences; and apply punctuation therein with informed confidence.

Rules & Exceptions

Terminal Punctuation

periods
Periods are most commonly used to mark closure. They may also be used as a mark of separation. Place a period at the end of a declarative sentence.

> **The patient's past medical history is unremarkable.**

Place a period at the end of an imperative sentence that does not require emphasis. For emphasis, use an exclamation point.

> **Do not lift heavy objects.**
> **Never lift heavy objects!**

Do not use a period at the end of a parenthetical sentence within another sentence.

> **When I saw him on his return visit (Dr. Smith saw him on his initial visit), I was startled by the deterioration in his condition.**

If a sentence terminates with an abbreviation (or other word) that ends with a period, do not add another period to end the sentence.

> **He takes Valium 5 mg q.a.m.**
>
> *not*
>
> **He takes Valium 5 mg q.a.m..**

Always place the period inside quotation marks.

> **The patient's response was emphatic: "I will never consent to the operation."**

In laboratory data, separate values of unrelated tests by periods.

> **White count 5.9. Urine specific gravity 1.006.**

question mark (?)

Direct inquiries. A question mark is used to indicate a direct inquiry. Thus, it is used at the end of an interrogative sentence (a direct question).

> **Was the patient seen in the emergency room prior to admission?**

Indirect questions. Use a period instead of a question mark at the end of indirect questions.

> **The patient asked if he could be discharged by Saturday.**

Sentences including the word *question*. Use a period instead of a question mark at the end of a declarative sentence that includes the word *question*.

> **I question the consultant's conclusions.**

Polite requests. Use a period instead of a question mark to end polite requests cast in the form of a question.

> **Would you please change my appointment to Saturday.**

Questions in the form of declarative statements. Place a question mark at the end of a question in the form of a declarative statement.

> **You mean you were serious when you said you smoke 50 cigarettes a day?**

Questions within declarative sentences. Place a question mark at the end of a question that is part of a declarative sentence.

> **How long will the operation take? we wondered.**

Series of incomplete questions. Place a question mark after each in a series of incomplete questions that immediately follow and relate to a preceding complete question.

> **When was the patient last seen? Friday? Saturday? Sunday?**

Expressions of doubt or uncertainty. Use an ending question mark to indicate doubt or uncertainty.

Sometimes, particularly with diagnoses, a question mark is placed before a statement in order to indicate uncertainty.

Placement either before or after the questionable material is acceptable, but do not place the question mark both before and after.

> His cholesterol levels were high normal (or mini-mally elevated?).
>
> DICTATED
> Diagnosis: Angina question mark
>
> TRANSCRIBED
> Diagnosis: Angina?
>
> *or*
>
> Diagnosis: ?Angina.
>
> *not*
>
> Diagnosis: ?Angina?
>
> Note: There is no space after the question mark in *?Angina*.

With other punctuation. Place the question mark inside the ending quotation mark if the material being quoted is in the form of a question. Follow *she said* or similar attributions with a comma when they precede a quoted question.

> The patient asked, "Must I return for followup that soon?"

Place the question mark outside the ending quotation mark if the quoted matter is not itself a question but is placed within an interrogative sentence.

> Do you think he meant it when he said, "You'll be hearing from my attorney"?

Never combine a question mark with a comma, or with another ending punctuation mark, i.e., an exclamation point, period, or other question mark. Thus, the question mark replaces the comma that normally precedes the ending quotation mark, which is followed by "he said" or similar attributions.

> **"Are my symptoms serious?" she asked.**

Place the question mark inside the closing parenthesis when the parenthetical matter is in the form of a question.

> **She said (did I hear correctly?) that she had 5 children, all delivered at home, and this is her first hospital admission.**

Place the question mark outside the closing parenthesis when the parenthetical matter occurs just prior to the end of an interrogative sentence but is not itself in the form of a question.

> **Did he return as scheduled for followup (the record is unclear)?**

exclamation point (!)

Use an exclamation point to express great surprise, incredulity, or other forceful emotion or comment. Use it primarily in direct quotations; avoid it otherwise in medical transcription except in rare instances. Use a comma or period for mild exclamations.

> **The patient loudly insisted, "You have already examined me!"**
> **"No," I replied quietly but firmly.**

Place the exclamation point inside the ending quotation mark if the material being quoted is an exclamatory statement. Never combine the exclamation point with a period, comma, question mark, or other exclamation point.

> **"Stop!" the patient cried as I approached her with the needle and syringe.**
>
> *not*
>
> **"Stop!," the patient cried . . .**

12|4

> **The patient insisted, "You have already examined me!"**
>
> *not*
>
> **The patient insisted, "You have already examined me!".**

Place the exclamation point before the closing parenthesis when an exclamatory statement is placed within parentheses.

> **The patient insisted I had already examined her (I had not!) and refused to cooperate.**

Place the exclamation point outside the closing parenthesis when the entire sentence (not just the parenthetical matter) is an exclamation.

> **What a fiasco (the patient left before I finished my exam)!**

Internal Punctuation

commas

Use a comma to indicate a break in thought, to set off material, and to introduce a new but connected thought.

Sometimes a comma must be used; sometimes it must not be used; sometimes its use is optional. Use commas when the rules require them and when they enhance clarity, improve readability, or diminish confusion or misunderstanding. Avoid their overuse.

Adjectives. Use commas to separate two or more adjectives if each modifies the noun alone.

> **Physical exam reveals a pleasant, cooperative, slender lady in no acute distress.**

Use commas to set off an adjective or adjectival phrase directly following the noun it modifies.

> **He has degenerative arthritis, left knee, with increasing inability to cope.**

HINT: If you can replace the comma between adjectives with *and*, the comma is necessary.

Appositives. Use commas before and after nonessential (or parenthetical) appositives.

> **The surgeons, Dr. Jones and Dr. Smith, reported that the procedure was a success.**

Conjunctions. Use a comma to separate independent clauses joined by a conjunction.

> **A consultation was obtained, and liver function studies were done.**

Coordinating conjunctions. Place a comma before a coordinating conjunction.

> **He was seen in the emergency room, but he was not admitted.**

Subordinating conjunctions. Place a comma before a subordinating conjunction in most cases.

> **He was in great pain, yet he refused treatment.**

However. Place a semicolon before and a comma after *however* when it is used as a conjunctive adverb, connecting two complete, closely related thoughts in a single sentence.

> **He is improved; however, he cannot be released.**

Place a comma after *however* when it serves as a bridge between two sentences.

> **The patient was released from care. However, his wife called to say his condition had worsened again.**

When *however* occurs in the second sentence and is not the first word, it is called an interruptive and requires a comma before and after it (unless it appears at the end of the sentence).

> DICTATED & TRANSCRIBED
> **He is improved. He cannot, however, be released.**
> **He is improved. He cannot be released, however.**

Dates. When the month, day, and year are given in this sequence, set off the year by commas.

> **She was admitted on December 14, 2001, and discharged on January 4, 2002.**

Genetics. Place a comma (without spacing) between the chromosome number and the sex chromosome. Use a virgule to indicate more than one karyotype in an individual.

> **The normal human karyotypes are 46,XX (female) and 46,XY (male).**

Geographic names. In text, use a comma before and after the state name preceded by a city name, or a country name preceded by a state or city name.

> **The patient moved to Modesto, California, 15 years ago.**
> **The patient returned from a business trip to Paris, France, the week prior to admission.**

Lists and series. Lists can take many forms. One style is a run-on (horizontal, narrative) list that uses commas or semicolons between items in the list.

> **He was sent home on Biaxin 500 mg b.i.d., Atrovent inhaler 2 puffs q.i.d., and Altace 5 mg daily.**
> **Her past history includes (1) diabetes mellitus, (2) cholecystitis, (3) hiatal hernia.**

Using a final comma before the conjunction preceding the last item in a series is optional unless its presence or absence changes the meaning.

> **Ears, nose, and throat are normal.** *(final comma optional)*
> **No dysphagia, hoarseness, or enlargement of the thyroid gland.** *(final comma required)*
> **The results showed blood sugar 46%, creatinine and BUN normal.** *(no comma after creatinine)*

Parenthetical expressions. Set off parenthetical expressions by commas.

> **A great deal of swelling was present, more so on the left than on the right.**

Use a comma before and after Latin abbreviations (and their translations), such as *etc., i.e., e.g., et. al., viz.,* when they are used as parenthetical expressions within a sentence.

> **Her symptoms come on with exertion, for example, when climbing stairs or running.**
> **Her symptoms come on with exertion, e.g., when climbing stairs or running.**

Quotation marks. Always place the comma following a quotation inside the closing quotation mark.

> **The patient stated that "the itching is driving me crazy," and she scratched her arms throughout our meeting.**

Titles. Lowercase job titles that are set off from a name by commas.

> **The pathology department secretary, John Smith, called us with the preliminary report.**

Units of measure. Do not use a comma or other punctuation between units of the same dimension.

> **The infant weighed 5 pounds 3 ounces.**

colon

The primary function of a colon as a punctuation mark is to introduce what follows: a list, series, or enumeration; an example; and sometimes a quotation (instead of a comma). Use either a single character space or two spaces following a colon, depending on your department or company policy for spacing at the end of a sentence; be consistent.

> **She said: "I have never gotten along with my mother, and I no longer try."**
>
> *or*
>
> **She said, "I have never gotten along with my mother, and I no longer try."**

Do not use a colon to introduce words that fit properly into the grammatical structure of the sentence without the colon, for example, after a verb, between a preposition and its object, or after *because.*

> **The patient is on Glucophage, furosemide, and Vasotec. (No colon after *on*)**
> **He came to the emergency room because he was experiencing fever and chills of several hours' duration. (No colon after *because*)**
>
> **HEENT: PERRLA, EOMI.**
>
> *or*

> **HEENT shows PERRLA, EOMI.**
>
> *not*
>
> **HEENT shows: PERRLA, EOMI.**

Capitalize the word following the colon if it is normally capitalized, if it follows a section or subsection heading, or if the list or series that follows the colon includes one or more complete sentences. Lowercase the first letter of each item in a series following a colon when the items are separated by commas.

> **The patient is on the following medications: Prevacid, prednisone, Bronkometer.**
>
> **ABDOMEN: Benign.**
> **Pelvic examination revealed the following: Moderately atrophic vulva. Markedly atrophic vaginal mucosa.**
>
> *or*
>
> **Pelvic examination revealed the following: moderately atrophic vulva, markedly atrophic vaginal mucosa.**
>
> *or*
>
> **Pelvic examination revealed moderately atrophic vulva, markedly atrophic vaginal mucosa.** *(no colon required)*

A colon may be used instead of a semicolon to separate two main clauses when the second one explains or expands upon the first.

> **He had numerous complaints; several were inconsistent with one another.**
>
> *or*

> **He had numerous complaints: several were inconsistent with one another.**

The colon is also used in numeric expressions of equator readings, ratios, and time. A colon may introduce a series or follow a heading or subheading, and it may replace a dash in some instances.

> **Sclerotomy drainage was done at the 8:30 equator.**

Formats. When the information following the section or subsection heading continues on the same line, use a colon (not a hyphen or a dash) after each heading.

> **HEENT: Within normal limits.**
> **THORAX AND LUNGS: No rales or rhonchi.**
> **CARDIOVASCULAR: No murmurs.**

Ratios. Express the value with numerals separated by a colon. Do not replace the colon with a virgule, dash, hyphen, or other mark.

> **Mycoplasma 1:2**
> **cold agglutinins 1:4**
> **Zolyse 1:10,000**
> **Xylocaine with epinephrine 1:200,000**

semicolons   In general, use a semicolon to mark a separation when a comma is inadequate and a period is too final.

Independent clauses. Use a semicolon to separate closely related independent clauses when they are not connected by a conjunction (*and, but, for, nor, yet, so*). Alternatively, the independent clauses may be written as separate sentences, but keep in mind that the semicolon demonstrates a relationship or link between the independent clauses that the period does not.

> **The patient had a radical mastectomy for a malignancy of the breast; the nodes were negative. (preferred)**
>
> **or**
>
> **The patient had a radical mastectomy for a malignancy of the breast. The nodes were negative. (acceptable)**

Use a semicolon before a conjunction connecting independent clauses if one or more of the clauses contain complicating internal punctuation.

> **The left inguinal region was prepped and draped in the usual fashion; and with 2% lidocaine for local anesthesia, a radiopaque #4-French catheter was introduced into the left common femoral artery, employing the Seldinger technique.**

Use a semicolon to separate closely related independent clauses when the second begins with a transitional word or phrase, such as *also, besides, however, in fact, instead, moreover, namely, nevertheless, rather, similarly, therefore, then,* or *thus.* Alternatively, the independent clauses may be written as separate sentences, but again, keep in mind that the semicolon shows a link or relationship between the clauses that the period does not.

> **The patient had a radical mastectomy for a malignancy of the breast; however, the nodes were negative. (preferred)**
>
> **or**
>
> **The patient had a radical mastectomy for a malignancy of the breast. However, the nodes were negative. (acceptable)**

Items in a series. Use a semicolon to separate items in a series if one or more items in the series include internal commas. This usage is frequently seen in lists of medications and dosages, as well as in lists of lab results.

> **The patient received Cerubidine 120 mg daily 3 times on February 26, 27, and 28, 2002; he received Cytosar 200 mg IV over 12 hours for 14 doses beginning February 26; and thioguanine 80 mg in the morning and 120 mg in the evening for 14 doses, for a total dose of 200 mg a day, starting February 26.**
> **His lab results showed white count 5.9, hemoglobin 14.6, hematocrit 43.1; PT 11.2, PTT 31.4; and urine specific gravity 1.006, pH 6, with negative dipstick and negative microscopic exam.**

Quotations. Always place the semicolon outside the quotation marks.

> **The patient clearly stated "no allergies"; yet, his medical record states he is allergic to penicillin.**

The Final Word

One important warning about applying punctuation should be heeded. If you find that you are having difficulty determining the appropriate punctuation for a dictated sentence, chances are the sentence is improperly constructed. Where gentle editing is permitted in a work setting, consider recasting the sentence in a way that preserves meaning but results in a construction that you can punctuate with confidence. Where editing is not permitted, there will be times when you may be unsure of how to salvage the sentence; however, keep in mind that some sentences just cannot be saved by punctuation.

Test Your Knowledge

Correctly punctuate the sentences below.

1. DIAGNOSIS: Fracture right leg.

2. She has a right-sided hemiparesis atrial fibrillation and diabetes.

3. After eating oysters at a party two days ago she began to get some bowel distention and this has rapidly increased today.

4. Because he became combative violent and abusive Security had to be involved in subduing the patient and haloperidol 5 mg and Ativan 2 mg IM was used to help control the patient.

5. Because of heavy bleeding that has repeatedly decreased the hematocrit to the 26% to 28% range and which interferes with the quality of life and ability to work the patient has requested TAH which will be carried out at this time.

6. Examination of the left lower extremity reveals 1+ swelling however there is no dependent edema present on examination.

7. RECOMMENDATION: Hydration analgesia observation and if stone does not pass within 72 hours or less will probably recommend the patient for ureteroscopy stone-basketing and ultrasonic lithotripsy.

8.   When asked if she had a history of drug abuse she replied Are you kidding?

9.   At the present time there is no nodule irregularity or active lesion and the biopsy site is well healed.

10.   SOCIAL HISTORY: The patient has two daughters one of whom is present with her today a son who lives out of state and two sisters who are alive and live close by.

Test Your Knowledge

Answers

1. DIAGNOSIS: Fracture, right leg.

2. She has a right-sided hemiparesis, atrial fibrillation, and diabetes.

3. After eating oysters at a party 2 days ago, she began to get some bowel distention, and this has rapidly increased today.

4. Because he became combative, violent, and abusive, Security had to be involved in subduing the patient, and haloperidol 5 mg and Ativan 2 mg IM were (*or* was) used to help control the patient.
    Note: The verb "was" is offered as an optional answer here, as these two drugs are typically administered in a single IM injection, necessitating them to be treated as unit, and thus a singular subject.

5. Because of heavy bleeding that has repeatedly decreased the hematocrit to the 26% to 28% range, and which interferes with the quality of life and ability to work, the patient has requested TAH, which will be carried out at this time.

6. Examination of the left lower extremity reveals 1+ swelling; however, there is no dependent edema present on examination.

7. RECOMMENDATION: Hydration, analgesia, observation, and if stone does not pass within 72 hours or less,

will probably recommend the patient for ureteroscopy, stone-basketing, and ultrasonic lithotripsy.

8. When asked if she had a history of drug abuse, she replied, "Are you kidding?"

9. At the present time there is no nodule, irregularity, or active lesion, and the biopsy site is well healed.

10. SOCIAL HISTORY: The patient has two daughters, one of whom is present with her today; a son who lives out of state; and two sisters who are alive and live close by.

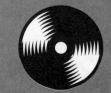

APPLICATION TEST
Take the application test for this chapter on your CD-ROM.
Access the section for
Chapter 12: "Punctuation."

Hyphens and Compound Modifiers

BOS Statement

Where?
BOS p. 91

A compound modifier consists of two or more words that act as a unit modifying a noun or pronoun. The use of hyphens to join these words varies depending on the type of compound modifier.

According to *The Gregg Reference Manual,* a modifier is *a word, phrase, or clause that qualifies, limits, or restricts the meaning of a word.* Healthcare documentation is a descriptive business. The accurate recording of a patient's care is often reliant on words and phrases that qualify, limit, or restrict the meaning of other words. As discussed in previous chapters, a patient's information—i.e., symptoms, complaints, diagnosis, etc.—has very little meaning unless fully qualified and/or quantified. A record that reflects that a patient presented to the emergency room with vaginal bleeding is not nearly as descriptive or diagnostically beneficial as one that indicates the patient presented with *profuse* vaginal bleeding, *scant* vaginal bleeding, or *mild-to-moderate* vaginal bleeding.

Nouns can have a single modifier (*scant* bleeding), they can have a string of separate modifiers (*thick, yellow* mucus), or they can have a modifier comprised of two or more words which alone do not modify the noun but when joined form a unique adjective (*mild-to-moderate* pain). In this last instance, the pain is neither mild nor moderate but somewhere in between. When two or more words combine to form a single modifier, or description, the resulting entity is called a *compound modifier* (sometimes called a *compound adjective*).

These unique adjectives are typically linked together by a hyphen. Occasionally in the evolution of language, that term will drop its hyphen and become a compound word. Most compound modifiers retain their hyphenation, however.

Going Deeper

Recognizing a compound modifier in dictation and applying the rules for hyphenation of those modifiers will require a sound understanding of parts of speech. You will note that many of the rules for compound modifiers provided in this chapter depend on the part of speech of each word and where the modifier occurs in relation to the noun it modifies. If you are unsure whether the two words in a compound construction represent an adjective-noun modifier (*third-story* window) or a noun-adjective modifier (*drug-dependent* patient), you will not be able to apply the correct rule for hyphenation (one of those constructions only takes a hyphen if it precedes the noun it modifies but not when it follows it).

A thorough review of parts of speech, particularly the role and function of a participle, will assist you in learning and understanding the compound modifier rules. While most of the time the inclusion or omission of a hyphen will not impact medical meaning, and would thus not be considered a critical error, occasionally the omission of a hyphen in a compound modifier *can* alter the meaning. For example, the meaning of the phrase *small-bowel obstruction* (an obstruction of the small bowel) would be greatly altered if it were not treated as a compound. *Small bowel obstruction* would imply that the *obstruction* was small, rather than identifying an obstruction of the *small bowel*.

The rest of the rules for hyphenation have been included in this chapter along with those related to compound words and compound modifiers. You should be familiar with those as well.

Rules & Exceptions

Compound Modifiers

Some compound modifiers are so commonly used together, or are so clear, that they are automatically read as a unit and do not need to be joined with hyphens.

> **dark brown lesion**
> **deep tendon reflexes**
> **1st trimester bleeding**
> **jugular venous distention**
> **left lower quadrant**
> **low back pain**
> **3rd degree burn**

adjective ending in –ly | Use a hyphen in a compound modifier beginning with an adjective that ends in -ly. (This requires distinguishing between adjectives ending in -ly and adverbs ending in -ly.) Do not use a hyphen with compound modifiers containing an adverb ending in -ly.

> **scholarly-looking patient**
>
> *but*
>
> **quickly paced steps**

adjective-noun compound | Use a hyphen in an adjective-noun compound that precedes and modifies another noun. *See:* noun-adjective compound on p. 236.

> **second-floor office**
>
> *but*
>
> **The office is on the second floor.**

233

adjective with preposition	Use hyphens in most compound adjectives that contain a preposition.

> **finger-to-nose test**

adjective with participle	Use a hyphen to join an adjective to a participle, whether the compound precedes or follows the noun.

> **good-natured, soft-spoken patient**
> **The patient is good-natured and soft-spoken.**

adverb with participle or adjective	Use a hyphen to form a compound modifier made up of an adverb coupled with a participle or adjective when the modifier precedes the noun it modifies but not when the modifier follows the noun.

> **well-developed and well-nourished woman**
>
> *but*
>
> **The patient was well developed and well nourished.**
> **fast-acting medication**
>
> *but*
>
> **The medication is fast acting.**

adverb ending in -*ly*	Do not use a hyphen in a compound modifier to link an adverb ending in -*ly* with a participle or adjective.

> **recently completed workup**
> **moderately acute pain**
> **financially stable investment**

adverb preceding a compound modifier	Do not use a hyphen in a compound modifier preceded by an adverb.

> **somewhat well nourished patient**

very

Drop the hyphen in a compound modifier with a participle or adjective when it is preceded by the adverb *very*.

> **very well developed patient**

disease-entity modifiers

Do not use hyphens with most disease-entity modifiers even when they precede the noun. Check appropriate medical references for guidance.

> **cervical disk disease**
> **oat cell carcinoma**
> **pelvic inflammatory disease**
> **sickle cell disease**
> **urinary tract infection**
> *but* **insulin-dependent diabetes mellitus and non-insulin-dependent diabetes mellitus**

eponyms

Use a hyphen to join two or more eponymic names used as multiple-word modifiers of diseases, operations, procedures, instruments, etc.

Do not use a hyphen if the multiple-word, eponymic name refers to a single person.

Use appropriate medical references to differentiate.

> **Osgood-Schlatter disease *(named for US orthopedic surgeon Robert B. Osgood and Swiss surgeon Carl Schlatter)*
> Chevalier Jackson forceps *(named for Chevalier Jackson, US pioneer in bronchoesophagology)***

equal, complementary, or contrasting adjectives

Use a hyphen to join two adjectives that are equal, complementary, or contrasting when they precede or follow the noun they modify.

> **anterior-posterior infarction**
> **physician-patient confidentiality issues**
> **His eyes are blue-green.**

foreign expressions

Do not hyphenate foreign expressions used in compound adjectives, even when they precede the noun they modify (unless they are always hyphenated).

> **in vitro experiments**
> **carcinoma in situ**
> **cul-de-sac** *(always hyphenated)*
> **ex officio member**

high- and low-

Use a hyphen in most *high-* and *low-* compound adjectives.

> **high-density mass**
> **low-frequency waves**
> **high-power field**

noun-adjective compound

Use a hyphen to join some noun-adjective compounds (but not all). Check appropriate references (dictionaries and grammar books).

When a hyphen is appropriate, use it whether the noun-adjective compound precedes or follows the noun it is modifying.

> **It is a medication-resistant condition.**
>
> *or*
>
> **The condition was medication-resistant.**
> **This is a symptom-free patient.**
>
> *or*
>
> **The patient was symptom-free.**
> **Stool is heme-negative.**

noun with participle	Use a hyphen to join a noun and a participle to form a compound modifier whether it comes before or after a noun.

> **bone-biting forceps**
> **She was panic-stricken.**
> **mucus-coated throat** *(the throat was coated with mucus, not mucous)*
> **callus-forming lesion** *(the lesion was forming callus, not callous)*

numerals with words	Use a hyphen between a number and a word forming a compound modifier preceding a noun.

> **3-week history**
> **2-year 5-month-old child**
> **8-pound 5-ounce baby girl**

proper nouns as adjective	Do not use hyphens in proper nouns even when they serve as a modifier preceding a noun.

> **John F. Kennedy High School**
> **New Mexico residents**

Do not use hyphens in combinations of proper noun and common noun serving as a modifier.

> **Tylenol capsule administration**

series of hyphenated compound modifiers	Use a suspensive hyphen after each incomplete modifier when there is a series of hyphenated compound modifiers with a common last word that is expressed only after the final modifier in the series.

> **10- to 12-year history**
> **full- and split-thickness grafts**

If one or more of the incomplete modifiers is not hyphenated, repeat the base with each, hyphenating or not, as appropriate.

> **preoperative and postoperative diagnoses (*not* pre- and postoperative diagnoses)**

to clarify or to avoid confusion

Use a hyphen to clarify meaning and to avoid confusion, absurdity, or ambiguity in compound modifiers. The hyphen may not be necessary if the meaning is made clear by the surrounding context.

> **large-bowel obstruction (obstruction of the large bowel, *not* a large obstruction of the bowel)**

hyphenated compound modifiers

Use a hyphen or en dash to join hyphenated compound modifiers or a hyphenated compound modifier with a one-word modifier.

> **non-disease-entity modifier**
>
> *or*
>
> **non–disease-entity modifier**

Use a hyphen or en dash to join two unhyphenated compound modifiers.

> **the North Carolina-South Carolina border**
>
> *or*
>
> **the North Carolina–South Carolina border**

Use a hyphen or en dash to join an unhyphenated compound modifier with a hyphenated one.

> **beta-receptor-mediated response (*or* β-receptor-mediated response)**
> ***or* beta-receptor–mediated response (*or* β-receptor–mediated response)**

Use a hyphen or en dash to join an unhyphenated compound modifier with a one-word modifier.

13|4

> **vitamin D-deficiency rickets**
> *or* **vitamin D–deficiency rickets**

Compound Words

Compound words may be written as one or multiple words; check dictionaries, grammar books, and other appropriate references.

hyphens

Hyphens are always used in some compound words, sometimes used in others, and never used in still others. Check dictionaries and other appropriate references for guidance.

> **attorney at law**
> **beta-blocker**
> **chief of staff**
> **father-in-law**
> **half-life**
> **near-syncope**
> **vice president**

Use a hyphen to join two nouns that are equal, complementary, or contrasting.

> **blood-brain barrier**
> **fracture-dislocation**

Do not hyphenate proper nouns of more than one word, even when they serve as a modifier preceding a noun.

> **South Dakota residents**

Do not use a hyphen in a combination of proper noun and common noun.

> **Tylenol capsule administration**

Use a hyphen with all compound nouns containing *ex-* when *ex-* means former and precedes a noun that can stand on its own.

> **ex-wife**
> **ex-president**

Use a hyphen in compound verbs unless one of the terms is a preposition.

> **single-space**
>
> *but*
>
> **follow up**

Sometimes hyphenated compound words become so well established that the hyphen is dropped and the words are joined together without a hyphen. When such a word can be used as *either* a noun, adjective, or verb, the noun and adjective forms are joined without a hyphen, but the verb form remains two separate words if one of them is a preposition.

noun, adjective	verb
checkup	check up
followup	follow up
workup	work up
followthrough	follow through

The patient was lost to followup. *(noun)*
Followup exam will be in 3 weeks. *(adjective)*
I will follow up the patient in 3 weeks. *(verb)*

HINT: To test whether the correct form is one word or two, try changing the tense or number. If one or more letters must be added, the correct form is two words.

> **We will follow up.**
> **tense change >>**
> **We followed up.**
> **(Followedup** *is not a word, so* **followed up** *must be two words.)*

> **We follow up.**
> **number change >>**
> **He follows up.**
> **(Followsup** *is not a word, so* **follows up** *must be two words.*)

Some terms consisting of a word followed by a single letter or symbol are hyphenated; others are not. Check appropriate references for guidance.

> **type 1 diabetes**
> **vitamin D**
> **Dukes A carcinoma**

Some terms with a single letter or symbol followed by a word are hyphenated, others are not. Check appropriate references for guidance, and consider the use of hyphens in such terms as optional if you are unable to document. Even if such terms are unhyphenated in their noun form, they should be hyphenated in their adjective form.

> **B-complex vitamins**
> **T wave**
> **T-wave abnormality**
> **x-rays**
> **x-ray results**

When a Greek letter is part of the name, use a hyphen after the symbol but not after the spelled-out form.

> **β-carotene** *but* **beta carotene**

plurals   For those written as a single word, form the plural by adding s.

> **fingerbreadths**
> **tablespoonfuls**
> **workups**

For those formed by a noun and modifier(s), form the plural by making the noun plural.

> **sisters-in-law**

For plural compound nouns containing a possessive, make the second noun plural.

> **associate's degrees**
> **driver's licenses**

For some compound nouns, the plural is formed irregularly.

> **forget-me-nots**

possessive forms

Use *'s* after the last word in a hyphenated compound term.

> **daughter-in-law's inquiry**

Hyphens

Hyphens as word connectors or joiners may be permanent or temporary. Over time, hyphenated terms may be replaced with the solid form. Check appropriate English and medical dictionaries for guidance.

Do not space before or after a hyphen with the exception of suspensive hyphens. *See:* suspensive hyphens on the next page.

clarity

Use hyphens to avoid confusion in meaning.

> **re-create (make again)** *not* **recreate (play)**
> **re-cover (cover again)** *not* **recover (from illness)**
> **re-place (put back in place)** *not* **replace (provide a substitute)**

Use hyphens to assist in pronunciation.

co-workers
re-study

suspensive hyphens

Single-space after a suspensive hyphen (one used to connect a series of compound modifiers with the same base term).

> **We used 3- and 4-inch bandages.**

We do not recommend using what might be called a "suspensive" hyphen in an expression such as *intra- and extrahepatic ducts*; rather, we would write out both words in full: *intrahepatic and extrahepatic ducts*.

vowel strings

Sometimes, use a hyphen to break up a string of three or more vowels, but other times do not; again, a dictionary should be your guide.

> **ileo-ascending**
>
> *but*
>
> **radioactive**

missing letters or numbers

Use a double hyphen or dash to represent missing letters or numbers. Be sure to place a space after the double hyphen or dash used to represent the ending letters or numbers in a term.

> **The patient said, "What the h— did he think I would do?"**

telephone numbers

Use hyphens following the area code and prefix of a telephone number. Alternatively, the area code may be placed in parentheses. If an extension is given, it is common practice to label it *ext*.

> **209-555-9620, ext. 104**
> **(209) 555-9620, ext. 104**

ZIP codes   Use a hyphen between the first five and last four digits of a ZIP-plus-four code.

> **Modesto, CA 95354-0550**

numbers and letters

> **CIN-1** *or* **CIN grade 1**
> **ST-T segment**
> **Q-wave pathology**
> **3-0 suture material**
> **beta-2 globulin**
> **α-globulin**
> **α2-globulin**
> **non-A, non-B hepatitis**
> **HLA-B27**
> **C-section**
> **2-D echo**
> **Obstetric history: 4-2-2-4.**
> **gravida 3, 3-0-0-3**
> **C1-2 disk space**

in place of dash

> **The patient agreed to return tomorrow—if he felt like it.**

range

> **8-12 wbc**
> **The office is open 1–4 p.m.**

QUICK REVIEW

Compounds that always take a hyphen	Compounds that take a hyphen only when preceding the noun
adjective ending in –ly	adjective-noun
adjective with participle	adjective with preposition
eponyms of two or more names	adverb with participle or adjective
equal, complementary, or contrasting adjectives	numerals with words
noun-adjective	
noun with participle	

The Final Word

Modifiers, or adjectives, add color and depth to language. In a clinical setting they are necessary for creation of an accurate, detailed story of a patient care encounter. As a general rule of thumb, you should analyze any progression of modifying words preceding a noun to determine if those words individually modify the noun or if any or all of them modify the noun only when combined with each other.

Test Your Knowledge

Correct the hyphenation errors in the sentences below where needed.

1. She presented with a 3-4 week history of intermittent headaches.

2. I told her to take Tylenol for her low grade fever.

3. The pharmacist told him the medication could be sleep-inducing.

4. She had a very short-lived career as a dancer.

5. The patient is a lovely looking female.

6. Apparently she cares for her elderly hard of hearing mother.

7. This is a gravida-3, para-3 female in no distress.

8. DIAGNOSIS: Nonhodgkin lymphoma.

9. He presented status post MVA with a right tibia fibula fracture.

10. She has no history of hypo- or hyperglycemia.

Test Your Knowledge

Answers

1. She presented with a 3- to 4-week history of intermittent headaches.

2. I told her to take Tylenol for her low-grade fever.

3. The pharmacist told him the medication could be sleep-inducing. (*Correct as is*)

4. She had a very short lived career as a dancer.

5. The patient is a lovely-looking female.

6. Apparently she cares for her elderly hard-of-hearing mother.

7. This is a gravida-3, para-3 female in no distress. (*Correct as is*)

8. DIAGNOSIS: Non-Hodgkin lymphoma.

9. He presented status post MVA with a right tibia-fibula fracture.

10. She has no history of hypoglycemia or hyperglycemia.

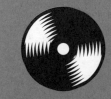

APPLICATION TEST
Take the application test for this chapter on your CD-ROM.
Access the section for
Chapter 13: "**Hyphens and Compound Modifiers.**"

Specialty Standards

Cardiology and Pulmonary Medicine

Heart disease continues to be the major cause of disability and death in the United States, and the recent focus on heart disease in women has brought even greater attention to the factors of lifestyle, genetics, diet, infection, and immunity in the diagnosis and treatment of cardiovascular disease. Cardiopulmonary medicine represents a core specialty in acute care. Patients present to and are admitted to the hospital for a wide variety of complex conditions, including hypertension, stroke, heart failure, cardiac arrhythmias, valvular heart disease, congenital heart disease, and pulmonary thromboembolism, the management of which involves a wide array of highly specialized radiologic and diagnostic procedures. Electrocardiography, vector cardiography, electrophysiologic studies, ultrasound, nuclear cardiology, radiology, catheterization, and pulmonary function testing are among these complex studies that an MT will encounter when transcribing in either the acute-care setting or in private practice. Since these conditions are common and so often chronic, the MT will encounter references to them and their related studies in almost every medical specialty.

Going Deeper

Given the fact that advancements in the treatment of cardiopulmonary disease are constantly emerging onto the clinical scene, medical transcriptionists need to have a particularly thorough understanding of this specialty in an acute-care setting. The standards that pertain to these two core areas focus primarily on the transcription of diagnostic testing and classification systems, but reference to these is common and students should leave the classroom equipped to encounter them in the healthcare documentation setting.

This chapter will orient you to the standards of style specific to the specialties of Cardiology and Pulmonary Medicine. Ideally, this section should be studied in conjunction with learning the anatomy, physiology, disease processes, etc., related to both of these complex specialties. Attempting to work through this chapter without a fundamental understanding of the body systems, conditions, symptoms, tests, and procedures related to these specialties could prove confusing and difficult. This chapter should also be coordinated with transcription application in these specialties so that the standards covered here can be reinforced through hands-on practice.

Rules & Exceptions

Cardiology

EKG terms   ECG and EKG are acceptable abbreviations for *electrocardiogram, electrocardiography, electrocardiographic*. Transcribe as dictated.

Leads. Electronic connections for recording by means of electrocardiograph. Where subscripts are called for but are not available, standard-size numerals and letters on the line may be used.

Standard bipolar leads. Use roman numerals.

> **lead I, lead II, lead III**

Augmented limb leads. Use a lowercase *a* followed by a capital *V*, then a capital *R* (right), *L* (left), or *F* (foot).

> **aVR, aVL, aVF**

Precordial leads. Use a capital *V* followed by an arabic numeral. Enter the numeral in the same point size on the line with the *V*, with no space between, or use subscripting.

> **V1, V2, V3, V4, V5, V6, V7, V8, V9**
>
> *or*
>
> **V$_1$, V$_2$, V$_3$, V$_4$, V$_5$, V$_6$, V$_7$, V$_8$, V$_9$**

Right precordial leads. Use a capital *V* followed by an arabic numeral and capital *R*. Enter the numeral and *R* in the same point size on the line with the *V*, with no space between, or use subscripting.

> **V3R, V4R, etc.**
>
> *or*
>
> **V$_3$R, V$_4$R, etc.**

Ensiform cartilage lead. Use a capital *V* followed by a capital *E* the same point size on the line with the *V*, with no space between, or subscript the *E*.

> **VE *or* V$_E$**

Third interspace leads. Use an arabic numeral followed by capital *V* and an arabic numeral. Enter the numeral following the *V* as a subscript or in the same point size on the line, with no space between.

> **3V1, 3V2, 3V3, etc.**
>
> *or*
>
> **3V$_1$, 3V$_2$, 3V$_3$, etc.**

Esophageal leads. Use a capital *E* followed by an arabic numeral either subscripted or on the line in the same point size, with no space between.

> **E15, E24, E50, etc.**
>
> *or*
>
> **E$_{15}$, E$_{24}$, E$_{50}$, etc.**

Sequential leads. Repeat the *V*. Do not use a hyphen or dash.

> **leads V1 through V5**
>
> *or*
>
> **V$_1$ through V$_5$**
>
> *not*
>
> **V1 through 5**
>
> *or*
>
> **V$_1$ through $_5$**
>
> *not*
>
> **V1-V5**
>
> *or*
>
> **V$_1$-V$_5$**
>
> *not*

V1-5

or

V$_{1-5}$

Tracing terms. In general, for electrocardiographic deflections, use all capitals, but larger and smaller *Q*, *R*, and *S waves* may be differentiated by capital and lower-case letters, respectively. Do not place a hyphen after the single letter except when the term is used as an adjective.

**Q wave, q wave
QS wave, qs wave
R wave, r wave
S wave, s wave
R' wave, r' wave (Note: R' is dictated as "R prime")
S' wave, s' wave**

For terms such as *P wave*, in which there is no hyphen, insert a hyphen when the term is used as an adjective (*P-wave pathology*).

**J junction
J point
P wave
QT interval, prolongation, etc.
QTc (*if subscript is not available, express as* QTc *or* corrected QT interval)
PR interval, segment, etc.
QRS axis, complex, configuration, etc.
ST segment
ST-T elevation
T wave
T-wave abnormality
Ta wave
U wave**

For *QRS axis*, use a plus or a minus sign followed by arabic numerals and a degree sign to express the number of degrees, e.g., *QRS +60°*, or write out *degrees: QRS +60 degrees*.

NOTE: There is no such thing as an ST wave or an ST-T wave, but it is common practice for providers to dictate the ST segment and the T wave together. Care should be taken to transcribe these references in a way that does not imply an ST wave or ST-T wave.

> DICTATED
> **STT wave abnormality**
>
> TRANSCRIBED
> **ST and T-wave abnormality**
> **ST-T-wave abnormality**
>
> *not*
>
> **STT-wave abnormality**
> **ST-T wave abnormality**

heart sounds and murmurs

Abbreviate heart sounds and components as follows, placing numerals on the line or using subscripts.

first heart sound	S1 *or* S_1
second heart sound	S2 *or* S_2
third heart sound	S3 *or* S_3
fourth heart sound	S4 *or* S_4
aortic valve component	A2 *or* A_2
mitral valve component	M1 *or* M_1
pulmonic valve component	P2 *or* P_2
tricuspid valve component	T1 *or* T_1

Express murmurs with arabic numerals 1 to 6 (from soft or low-grade to loud or high-grade). Do not use roman numerals. Murmurs are expressed on either a scale of 1 to 4 or a scale of 1 to 6. The scale of 6 breaks down as follows:

grade 1	barely audible, must strain to hear
grade 2	quiet, but clearly audible
grade 3	moderately loud
grade 4	loud
grade 5	very loud; audible with stethoscope partly off the chest
grade 6	so loud that it can be heard with stethoscope just above chest wall

Place a virgule between the murmur grade and the scale used (2/6 = a grade 2 murmur on a scale of 6).

> **grade 1/6 systolic murmur**

Express partial units as indicated.

> DICTATED
> **grade 4 and a half over 6 murmur**
>
> TRANSCRIBED
> **grade 4.5 over 6 murmur**
>
> *or*
>
> **grade 4.5/6 murmur**
>
> DICTATED
> **grade 4 to 5 over 6 murmur**
>
> TRANSCRIBED
> **grade 4 to 5 over 6 murmur**
>
> *or*
>
> **grade 4/6 to 5/6 murmur**
>
> *not*
>
> **grade 4-5/6 murmur**
>
> DICTATED
> **to-and-fro SDM**
>
> TRANSCRIBED
> **to-and-fro systolic-diastolic murmur**

A bruit is an abnormal heart sound or murmur heard on auscultation. The plural form is *bruits* but because of the French origin of the word, often the final *s* is not pronounced and the singular and plural forms sound the same: "*broo-ee.*"

Spell out the following abbreviations even when they are dictated in phonocardiographic tracings.

ASM	atrial systolic murmur
CM	continuous murmur
DM	diastolic murmur
DSM	delayed systolic murmur
ESM	ejection systolic murmur
IDM	immediate diastolic murmur
LSM	late systolic murmur
PSM	pansystolic murmur
SDM	systolic-diastolic murmur
SEM	systolic ejection murmur
SM	systolic murmur
AEC	aortic ejection click
AOC	aortic opening click
C	click
E	ejection sound
EC	ejection click
NEC	nonejection click
PEC	pulmonary ejection click
OS	opening snap
SC	systolic click
SS	summation sound
W	whoop

NYHA classi-fication of cardiac failure

Widely adopted classification of cardiac failure that was developed by the New York Heart Association. Lower-case *class*; use roman numerals I through IV.

I	asymptomatic
II	comfortable at rest, symptomatic with normal activity
III	comfortable at rest, symptomatic with less than normal activity
IV	severe cardiac failure, symptomatic at rest

DIAGNOSIS: **Cardiac failure, class III.**

pacemaker codes

Capitalize these three-letter codes, without spaces or periods.

AVD
ITR

First and second letters refer to:

A   atrium
V   ventricle
D   dual, both atrium and ventricle

Third letter refers to:

I   inhibited response
T   triggered response
R   rate-responsive response

TIMI system   Thrombolysis in myocardial infarction. A grading system (grade 0 to 3) for coronary perfusion; evaluates reperfusion achieved by thrombolytic therapy. Lowercase *grade* and use arabic numerals.

> **The patient had TIMI grade 3 flow at 90 minutes following thrombolytic therapy.**

Pulmonary and Respiratory Terms

breaths per minute, respirations per minute   Spell out. Do not abbreviate.

> **Respirations: 18 breaths per minute.**
>
> *not*
>
> **Respirations: 18 bpm.**
> **21 respirations per minute**
>
> *not*
>
> **21 rpm**

Use virgules only in the following form.

> **Respirations: 21/min**
>
> *not*
>
> **21 respirations/min**

primary symbols

Primary symbols used in pulmonary and respiratory terminology are the first terms of an expression and are expressed as follows.

C	**blood gas concentration**
P *or* p	**pressure or partial pressure**
Q	**volume of blood**
V	**volume of gas**
D	**diffusing capacity**
R	**gas exchange ratio**

secondary symbols for gas phase

Immediately follow the primary symbol. Express as small capitals if possible; otherwise, use regular caps.

A *or* A	**alveolar**
B *or* B	**barometric**
E *or* E	**expired**
I *or* I	**inspired**
L *or* L	**lung**
T *or* T	**tidal**

secondary symbols for blood phase

Immediately follow the secondary symbol for gas phase. Express as lowercase letters.

b	**blood**
a	**arterial**
c	**capillary**
v	**venous**

gas abbreviations

Usually the last element of the term. Express as small capitals or regular capitals. Use subscripts or place the numerals on the line.

CO2 *or* CO$_2$ *or* CO2
O2 *or* O$_2$ *or* O2
N2 *or* N$_2$ *or* N2
CO *or* CO

physiology terms

Combine the above symbols for pulmonary and respiratory physiology terms.

P CO$_2$ *or* pCO$_2$	partial pressure of carbon dioxide
PaCO$_2$	partial pressure of arterial carbon dioxide
P O$_2$ *or* pO$_2$	partial pressure of oxygen
PaO$_2$	partial pressure of arterial oxygen
V/Q	ventilation-perfusion ratio

The Final Word

Most MTs find cardiopulmonary studies and procedures to be fascinating, and it is little wonder that it is the most frequently sought after by MTs seeking to specialize. Rapid developments in cardiology have made it such a complex field that those who do specialize in it still find it challenging and rewarding even after years in the specialty, though certainly it is one that demands much from the MT in terms of continuing education. Whether it is the depth of anatomy found in cardiovascular surgery or the science of electrophysiology, you will find cardiopulmonary medicine a rich and diverse focus of study.

Test Your Knowledge

Correct the errors in each of the sentences below.

1. She had ST-segment depression in leads 2, 3 and AVL.

2. Examination revealed a positive grade II/VI systolic murmur.

3. The patient had T wave inversions in V-4 through V-6.

4. He has been following her for her class-2 cardiac failure.

5. Heart sounds are regular, with S-1 and S-2 normal.

6. There is a faint half over 6 systolic ejection murmur.

7. There is a diphasic T-wave in 2, 3, AVF, V5 and 6.

8. DIAGNOSIS: Status post implantation of AICD.

9. The ST segments are depressed in leads V1-6.

10. Arterial blood gases revealed Po2 and PCo2 to be within normal limits.

Test Your Knowledge

Answers

1. She had ST-segment depression in leads II, III and aVL.

2. Examination revealed a positive grade 2/6 systolic murmur.

3. The patient had T-wave inversions in V4 through V6.

4. He has been following her for her class II cardiac failure.

5. Heart sounds are regular, with S1 and S2 normal.

6. There is a faint 1/2 over 6 systolic ejection murmur.

7. There is a diphasic T wave in II, III, aVF, V5 and V6.

8. DIAGNOSIS: Status post implantation of automatic implantable cardioverter-defibrillator.

9. The ST segments are depressed in leads V1 through V6.

10. Arterial blood gases revealed PO_2 and PCO_2 to be within normal limits.

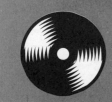

APPLICATION TEST
Take the application test for this chapter on your CD-ROM.
Access the section for
Chapter 14: "Cardiology and Pulmonary Medicine."

Hematology/ Oncology & Laboratory Medicine

Examinations performed on body fluids, such as blood, cerebrospinal fluid, waste products, and abnormal products (calculi, for example) are critical to the diagnosis and treatment of disease. Such examinations fall under a branch of pathology called clinical pathology that is focused on quantitative analysis in these areas. Anatomic pathology, on the other hand, deals with the gross and microscopic evaluation of living human tissue to determine the presence, extent and evolution of disease. Both branches are encountered constantly in healthcare documentation, both in the documentation of laboratory tests and values and the pathologic findings reported in multiple specialties, most specifically *oncology*.

Recognizing and applying standards that relate to laboratory medicine will require an in-depth understanding of blood and tissue anatomy, basic hematology and histology, and the disease process of malignancy. *The Book of Style* provides standards specific to the transcription of blood references, laboratory tests and values, and cancer medicine. Given the high degree of potential error associated with this area of a patient's report, transcriptionists are encouraged to be particularly vigilant in both preparation and application of these standards. The incorrect transcription or transposition of a lab name or value or an error in transcribing the classification of disease in an oncology report could carry potential for risk to the patient. This represents an area of the report where clarity and accuracy are crucial, and transcriptionists need to be extra cautious here.

Going Deeper

Laboratory medicine and oncology represent two areas where ongoing education is very important. Cutting-edge laboratory tests, particularly in the area of genetic research and genomics, are constantly emerging onto the scene of clinical practice and diagnostic application. New chemotherapy trials in oncology, new clinical trials for chronic diseases like HIV and hepatitis, and new tumor marker identifications can make this specialty a constant challenge for the MT who works in acute care or in the specialty of hematology/oncology.

This chapter will orient you to the standards of style specific to these areas. Ideally, this section should be studied in conjunction with learning the anatomy, physiology, disease processes, etc., related to these complex specialties. Attempting to work through this chapter without a fundamental understanding of the anatomy and physiology and disease processes related to these specialties could prove confusing and difficult. This chapter should also be coordinated with transcription application in these specialties so that the standards covered here can be reinforced through hands-on practice.

Rules & Exceptions

General Laboratory Data & Values

laboratory data and values

Use numerals to express laboratory values.

Punctuation. Do not use commas to separate a lab value from the test it describes.

> white count 5300
>
> *not*
>
> white count, 5300

When multiple lab results are given, separate related tests by commas. Use semicolons if entries in the series have internal commas.

> White count 5.9, hemoglobin 14.6, hematocrit 43.1.

Separate unrelated tests by periods. If uncertain whether tests are related or unrelated, use periods.

> White count 5.9, hemoglobin 14.6, hematocrit 43.1. Urine specific gravity 1.006, pH 6, negative dipstick.
> Blood work showed white count of 4800 with 58 segs, 7 bands, 24 lymphs, 8 monos, 2 eos, and 2 basos; hemoglobin 14.6 and hematocrit 43.1.

Electrolytes. Substances that dissociate into positive and negative ions in solution. The electrolytes generally include sodium, potassium, chloride, and total CO_2 or bicarbonate. Anion gap may also be reported.

Though not technically electrolytes, BUN, creatinine, and glucose are also part of a chemistry profile and often dictated in the same breath.

> **DIAGNOSTIC DATA**
>
> Electrolytes: Sodium 139, potassium 4.6, chloride 106, bicarb 28. BUN 15, creatinine 0.9, glucose 132. White count 5.9, hemoglobin 14.6, hematocrit 43.1.

Hemoglobin and hematocrit. Hemoglobin and hematocrit values are often dictated "H and H" or "H over H." For clarity, translate the abbreviations into their respective terms.

> DICTATED
> **H and H 11.8 and 35.3.**
>
> TRANSCRIBED
> **Hemoglobin 11.8 and hematocrit 35.3.**

Percentage values. Use the expression dictated.

> **MCHC 34%**
> *or* **MCHC 0.34**
> *or* **MCHC 34**
> **polys 58%**
> *or* **polys 0.58**
> *or* **polys 58**

Do not convert unless the forms are mixed; then make them consistent.

> DICTATED
> **White count was 4800 with 58 segs, 7 bands, 24 lymphs, 8 monos, 2% eos, and 2% basos.**
>
> TRANSCRIBED
> **White count was 4800 with 58 segs, 7 bands, 24 lymphs, 8 monos, 2 eos, and 2 basos.**

Specific gravity. Express with four digits and a decimal point placed between the first and second digits. Do not drop the final zero.

> DICTATED
> **Specific gravity ten twenty**
>
> TRANSCRIBED
> **Specific gravity 1.020**

Tumor cell markers. Express with capital letters and arabic numerals, without spaces or punctuation between letter and number.

> **CD4**
> **CD52**

Urinalysis. Term evolved from *urine analysis,* which is now archaic. Edit to *urinalysis.* Use abbreviation *UA* only if dictated.

> DICTATED
> **Urine analysis showed...**
>
> TRANSCRIBED
> **Urinalysis showed...**

Hematology

blood counts

Differential blood count. Part of a white blood cell count. Includes polymorphonuclear leukocytes (PMNs, polys, segmented neutrophils [segs]), band neutrophils (bands, stabs), lymphocytes (lymphs), eosinophils (eos), basophils (basos), and monocytes (monos).

Differential counts may be given as whole numbers or as percents; total should equal 100 in either case.

> **White blood count of 4800, with 58% segs, 7% bands, 24% lymphs, 8% monos, 1% eos, and 2% basos.**
>
> *or*
>
> **White blood count of 4800, with 58 segs, 7 bands, 24 lymphs, 8 monos, 1 eo, and 2 basos.**

RBC, rbc. Either form is acceptable as an abbreviation for red blood count or red blood cells.

WBC, wbc. Either form is acceptable as an abbreviation for white blood count or white blood cells.

blood groups

ABO system. Use single or dual letters, sometimes with a subscript letter or number. If subscripts are not available, place the numeral immediately following and on the line with the letter.

> **group A**
> **group A1 or group A_1**
> **group A1B or group A_1B**

Other systems. Other common blood group systems include Auberger, Diego, Duffy, Kell, Kidd, Lewis, Lutheran, Rh (not Rhesus), Sutter, and Xg. Consult laboratory references for guidance in expressing terms related to these and other blood groups.

blood types

Write out *B negative* or *B positive* rather than *B−* or *B+*, because the minus or plus sign is easily overlooked.

clotting factors

Lowercase *factor*. Use roman numerals.

> | | |
> |---|---|
> | **factor I** | **fibrinogen** |
> | **factor II** | **prothrombin** |
> | **factor III** | **thromboplastin** |
> | **factor IV** | **calcium ions** |
> | **factor V** | **proaccelerin** |
> | **factor VI** | **(none currently designated)** |
> | **factor VII** | **proconvertin** |
> | **factor VIII** | **antihemophilic factor** |
> | **factor IX** | **Christmas factor** |
> | **factor X** | **Stuart factor** |
> | **factor XI** | **plasma thromboplastin antecedent** |
> | **factor XII** | **glass factor** |
> | **factor XIII** | **fibrin-stabilizing factor** |

Platelet factors. Use arabic numerals for platelet factors (abbreviation: PF).

> **platelet factor 3**
> **PF 3 *(Note: Space between PF and the numeral.)***

Activated form. Add a lowercase *a* to designate a factor's activated form.

factor Xa

Von Willebrand (factor VIII). Newer terms for factor VIII (also known as von Willebrand factor) are preferred, but older terms continue to be used. Transcribe the dictated form, expressing it appropriately.

old term	newer term
factor VIII:C	factor VIII
factor VIII:CAg	factor VIII:Ag
von Willebrand factor	vWF
factor VIII:RAg	vWF Ag
VIII:RCoF	ristocetin cofactor

complement factors

Factors involved in antigen-antibody reactions and inflammation. Immediately follow a capital *C*, *B*, *P*, or *D* with an arabic numeral on the line.

C1
C7

Add a lowercase letter (usually *a* or *b*) for fragments of complement components.

C5a
Bb

globulins

Spell out English translations of Greek letters. Place the arabic numeral (if included) on the line and connect it to the English translation of the Greek letter with a hyphen. Use a character space before the word *globulin*.

beta globulin
beta-2 globulin

When using Greek letters, place a hyphen between the Greek letter (with or without subscript) and *globulin*.

β-globulin
β 2-globulin

Immunoglobulins are expressed as follows:

IgA
IgD
IgE
IgG
IgM

Gram stain   A method of differential staining of bacteria devised by Hans Gram, a Danish physician. Capitalize the *G* in *Gram stain*.

We ordered a Gram stain stat.

Lowercase *gram-negative* and *gram-positive*.

The specimen was gram-negative.
The culture grew out gram-positive cocci.

hepatitis
nomenclature   Use capital letters to designate type. Do not use a hyphen to connect the word *hepatitis* to the letter designating its type, but do use a hyphen to connect *non* to the letter.

hepatitis A
hepatitis C
non-A hepatitis
non-B hepatitis
non-A, non-B hepatitis
delta hepatitis

Related abbreviations:

HAV	**hepatitis A virus**
HBAg	**hepatitis B antigen**
HBsAg	**hepatitis B surface antigen**
HBIG	**hepatitis B immunoglobulin**
HBV	**hepatitis B virus**
anti-HAV	**antibody to hepatitis A**
anti-HBV	**antibody to hepatitis B**

Previous designations of viral hepatitis, such as infectious hepatitis, short-incubation-period hepatitis, long-incubation-period hepatitis, and serum hepatitis are no longer preferred but should be transcribed if dictated.

hormones

Hormones may be referred to by their therapeutic or diagnostic names, their native names, or their abbreviations. In abbreviated form, place numerals on the line or subscript.

therapeutic/diagnostic name	native name	abbreviation
chorionic gonadotropin	human chorionic gonadotropin	hCG
corticotropin, purified	corticotropin (*previously adrenocorticotropic hormone*)	ACTH
triiodothyronine	triiodothyronine	T3 *or* T_3
thyrotropin	thyroid-stimulating hormone	TSH
thyroxine	thyroxine	T4 *or* T_4

The preferred suffix is *-tropin* (indicating an ability to change or redirect), not *-trophic* (indicating a relationship to nutrition).

thyrotropin-releasing hormone
gonadotropin-releasing hormone
corticotropin
somatotropin

human leukocyte antigen (HLA)

Test that detects genetic markers on white blood cells. Abbreviation: HLA. Express with capital-lowercase combinations and hyphens. Check appropriate references for guidance.

HLA-DR5   **associated with Hashimoto thyroiditis**
B8, Dw3   **associated with Graves disease**

Major histocompatibility complex, class I antigens:

> **HLA-D**
> **HLA-DR**

Major histocompatibility complex, class II antigens:

> **HLA-B27**
> **HLA-DRw10**

Examples of antigenic specificities of major HLA loci:

> **HLA-A**
> **HLA-B**
> **HLA-C**
> **HLA-D**

lymphocytes T lymphocytes (T cells) and B lymphocytes (B cells) are the most common lymphocytes. T means thymus-derived, B means bursa-derived. In general, do not use the extended forms.

Hyphenation. Do not hyphenate except when used as an adjective preceding a noun.

> **T cells**
> **T-cell count**

Pre- and pan-. Use a hyphen to join *pre-* or *pan-* to the following letter or word.

> **pre-T cell**
> **pan-B lymphocyte**
> **pan-thymocyte**

Subsets of T lymphocytes. Use a virgule (not a hyphen) to express helper/inducer and cytotoxic/suppressor subsets of T lymphocytes.

Helper/inducer T lymphocytes are also known as helper cells or helper T lymphocytes.

Cytotoxic/suppressor T lymphocytes are also called suppressor cells.

Use a hyphen (not a virgule or colon) in the phrase *helper-suppressor ratio*.

> **helper-suppressor ratio**
> *not* **helper/suppressor ratio**
> *not* **helper:suppressor ratio**

Surface antigens. Join arabic numerals (on the line) to the letter *T* to express surface antigens of T lymphocytes.

> **T3**
> **T8**
> **T11**

Cancer Classifications

stage and grade

Lowercase *stage* and *grade*. Use roman numerals for cancer stages. For subdivisions of cancer stages, add capital letters on the line and arabic suffixes, without internal spaces or hyphens.

> **stage 0 (indicates carcinoma in situ)**
> **stage I, stage IA**
> **stage II, stage II3**
> **stage III**
> **stage IV, stage IVB**

Use arabic numerals for grades.

> **grade 1**
> **grade 2**
> **grade 3**
> **grade 4**

Aster-Coller: Staging system for colon cancer from the least involvement at stage A and B1 through the most extensive involvement at stage D.

> **The patient's Aster-Coller B2 lesion extends through the entire thickness of the colon wall, with no involvement of nearby nodes.**

Broders index: Classification of aggressiveness of tumor malignancy developed in the 1920s by AC Broders. Reported as grade 1 (most differentiation and best prognosis) through grade 4 (least differentiation and poorest prognosis). Lowercase *grade*; use arabic numerals.

> **Broders grade 3**

Cervical cytology. Three different systems are currently in use for cervical cytology: the Papanicolaou test (Pap smear), the CIN classification system, and the Bethesda system.

The Papanicolaou test uses roman numerals to classify cervical cytology samples from class I (within normal limits) through class V (carcinoma).

CIN is an acronym for cervical intraepithelial neoplasia and is expressed with arabic numerals from grade 1 (least severe) to grade 3 (most severe). Place a hyphen between CIN and the numeral.

> **CIN-1, CIN-2, CIN-3**
>
> *or*
>
> **CIN grade 1, CIN grade 2, CIN grade 3**

A cervical cytology sample that is within normal limits in the Bethesda system corresponds with a Pap class I or II; Bethesda's atypical squamous cell of undetermined significance (ASCUS) corresponds with Pap class III; Bethesda's low-grade squamous intraepithelial lesion (LGSIL) corresponds with Pap class III and CIN grade 1; and Bethesda's high-grade squamous intraepithelial lesion (HGSIL) corresponds with Pap classes III and IV and CIN grades 2 and 3. In the Bethesda system, the next higher level is labeled simply "carcinoma," corresponding with Pap class V and with "carcinoma" in the CIN system.

Clark level: Describes invasion level of primary malignant melanoma of the skin from the epidermis.

Use roman numerals I (least deep) to IV (deepest). Lowercase *level*.

Clark level I	**into underlying papillary dermis**
Clark level II	**to junction of papillary and reticular dermis**
Clark level III	**into reticular dermis**
Clark level IV	**into the subcutaneous fat**

Dukes classification: Named for British pathologist Cuthbert E. Dukes (1890-1977). Classifies extent of operable adenocarcinoma of the colon or rectum. Do not use an apostrophe before or after the *s*. Follow *Dukes* with capital letter.

Dukes A	**confined to mucosa**
Dukes B	**extending into the muscularis mucosae**
Dukes C	**extending through the bowel wall, with metastasis to lymph nodes**

When the Dukes classification is further defined by numbers, use arabic numerals on the same line with the letter, with no space between.

Dukes C2

FAB classification: French-American-British morphologic classification system for acute nonlymphoid leukemia. Express with capital *M* followed by arabic numeral (1 through 6); do not space between the *M* and the numeral.

M1	**myeloblastic, no differentiation**
M2	**myeloblastic, differentiation**
M3	**promyelocytic**
M4	**myelomonocytic**
M5	**monocytic**
M6	**rythroleukemia**

FAB staging of carcinoma utilizes TNM classification of malignant tumors (see: TNM staging below).

> **FAB T1 N1 M0**

FIGO staging: Federation Internationale de Gynécologie et Obstétrique system for staging gynecologic malignancy, particularly carcinomas of the ovary. Expressed as stage I (least severe) to stage IV (most severe), with subdivisions within each stage (a, b, c). Lowercase *stage*, and use roman numerals. Use lowercase letters to indicate subdivisions within a stage.

> **Diagnosis: Ovarian carcinoma, FIGO stage IIc.**

Gleason tumor grade: Also known as *Gleason score*. The system scores or grades the prognosis for adenocarcinoma of the prostate, with a scale of 1 through 5 for each dominant and secondary pattern; these are then totaled for the score. The higher the score, the poorer the prognosis. Lowercase *grade* or *score*, and use arabic numerals.

> **Diagnosis: Adenocarcinoma of prostate, Gleason score 8.**
> **Gleason score 3 + 2 = 5.**
> **Gleason 3 + 3 with a total score of 6.**

Jewett classification of bladder carcinoma: Use capitals as follows:

> | | |
> |---|---|
> | O | in situ (Note: this is the letter O, not a zero) |
> | A | involving submucosa |
> | B | involving muscle |
> | C | involving surrounding tissue |
> | D | involving distant sites |
>
> **Diagnosis: Bladder carcinoma, Jewett class B.**

Karnofsky rating scale, Karnofsky status: Scale for rating performance status of patients with malignant neoplasms. Use arabic numerals: 10, 20, 30, 40, 50, 60, 70, 80, 90, 100. (Normal is 100, moribund is 10.)

TNM staging system for malignant tumors:

System for staging malignant tumors, developed by the American Joint Committee on Cancer and the Union Internationale Contre le Cancer.

> T   **tumor size or involvement**
> N   **regional lymph node involvement**
> M   **extent of metastasis**

Write TNM expressions with arabic numerals on the line and a space after each number.

> **T2 N1 M1**
> **T4 N3 M1**

Letters and symbols following the letters *T*, *N*, and *M*:

> ***X* means assessment cannot be done.**
> ***0* (zero) indicates no evidence found.**
> **Numbers indicate increasing evidence of the characteristics represented by those letters.**
> ***Tis* indicates tumor in situ.**
> **Tis N0 M0**

The TNM system criteria for defining cancer stages vary according to the type of cancer. Thus a stage II cancer of one type may be defined as T1 N0 M0, while one of another type may be defined as T2 N1 M0.

Staging indicators are used along with TNM criteria to define cancers and assess stages. These are expressed with capital letters and arabic numerals.

> | | |
> |---|---|
> | **grade** | **GX, G1, G2, G3, G4** |
> | **host performance** | **H0, H1, H2, H3, H4** |
> | **lymphatic invasion** | **LX, L0, L1, L2** |
> | **residual tumor** | **RX, R0, R1, R2** |
> | **scleral invasion** | **SX, S0, S1, S2** |
> | **venous invasion** | **VX, V0, V1, V2** |

Prefixes. Lowercase prefixes on the line with *TNM* and other symbols indicate criteria used to describe and stage the tumor, e.g., *cTNM, aT2*.

letter	determining criteria
a	autopsy staging
c	clinical classification
P	pathological classification
r	retreatment classification
y, yp	classification during or following treatment with multiple modalities

Suffixes. The suffix *(m)* (in parentheses) indicates the presence of multiple primary tumors in a single site. Other suffixes may be used, such as the following in the nasopharynx:

T2a	nasopharyngeal tumor extending to soft tissues of oropharynx and/or nasal fossa *without* parapharyngeal extension
T2b	nasopharyngeal tumor extending to soft tissues of oropharynx and/or nasal fossa *with* parapharyngeal extension

The Final Word

This complex and detailed chapter is packed with new information that may seem overwhelming. Some of it may be encountered rarely in the course of your career, but it is more likely that you will hear most of it on a daily basis, particularly in acute care. While laboratory tests have historically been used primarily to diagnose disease, they are now used just as frequently to track the course or progress of a disease as well as the progress and efficacy of treatment. They are at the heart of diagnostic medicine and are fundamental to managing care for just about every patient in the healthcare system. A skilled MT will stay abreast of the trends and changes in these key areas in order to ensure cutting-edge accuracy in the healthcare record.

Test Your Knowledge

Correct the errors in each of the sentences below.

---

1. LABORATORY DATA: White count, 3300, with a normal differential.

2. Urine analysis showed a specific gravity of 10.20, with 3 to 4 WBC's per high power field.

3. She was found to have PT-1 PN-0 PM-X neuroblastoma.

4. The patient has Clark level 3 malignant melanoma.

5. I explained to the patient that a detectable antibody to HB-SAG would indicate immunity to hepatitis B.

6. IGa, IGe, and IGm were all within normal limits.

7. DIAGNOSIS: FIGO stage 2b ovarian carcinoma.

8. She did have a Pap last year that revealed CIN I neoplasia, but repeat Pap was normal.

9. He has Factor 5 Leiden thrombophilia, diagnosed in his early 30's.

10. We will be tracking the patient's helper-inducer T-cells closely.

Test Your Knowledge

Answers

1. LABORATORY DATA: White count 3300 with a normal differential.

2. Urinalysis showed a specific gravity of 1.020, with 3 to 4 WBCs (*or* wbc's) per high-power field.

3. She was found to have pT1 pN0 pMX neuroblastoma.

4. The patient has Clark level III malignant melanoma.

5. I explained to the patient that a detectable antibody to HBsAg would indicate immunity to hepatitis B.

6. IgA, IgE, and IgM were all within normal limits.

7. DIAGNOSIS: FIGO stage IIb ovarian carcinoma.

8. She did have a Pap last year that revealed CIN-1 neoplasia, but repeat Pap was normal.

9. He has Factor V Leiden thrombophilia, diagnosed in his early 30s.

10. We will be tracking the patient's helper/inducer T cells closely.

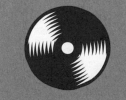

APPLICATION TEST
Take the application test for this chapter on your CD-ROM.
Access the section for
Chapter 15: "Hematology/Oncology & Laboratory Medicine."

16

Obstetrics, Gynecology & Genetics

Certainly few specialties are more enjoyable to allied health-care workers than obstetrics and gynecology. The areas of labor and delivery and neonatal intensive care are much sought after by many in the clinical setting. This is one of the few areas of the hospital where the majority of patients are happy to be there! Being a participant in the birth of a baby can be a rewarding branch of applied medicine. Medical transcriptionists likewise tend to enjoy the exposure to this specialty in the acute care setting, where a typical day for most hospital MTs will include a healthy mix of routine deliveries and C-sections. MTs are afforded a glimpse into the beginning of life for the next generation, and transcribing the birth of a healthy baby to parents plagued by years of infertility will always be a welcome joy, particularly after transcribing a report on a mother of two who has lost her battle to breast cancer.

Around this specialty of reproductive health, of course, exist the areas of gynecology, neonatology, and genetics. In the gynecologic setting, an MT will encounter terminology, tests, and diagnoses related to vaginal, cervical, and uterine health, as well as those that pertain to the ovulatory cycle, hormone regulation, and infertility. It is important to remember that this specialty also includes the evolving reproductive health of women as they approach and transition through menopause.

This chapter will orient you to the standards of style specific to these areas. Ideally, this section should be studied in conjunction with learning the anatomy, physiology, disease processes, etc., related to these complex specialties. Attempting to work through this chapter without a fundamental understanding of the anatomy and physiology and disease processes related to these specialties could prove confusing and difficult. This chapter should also be coordinated with transcription application in this area so that the standards covered here can be reinforced through hands-on practice.

Going Deeper

The identification and study of genetic abnormalities and defects has become an area of increased clinical focus over recent years. The applications of genetic research are far-reaching, and significant research into the cause and cure of most major diseases and illnesses today is being directed at genomics, which is focused on manipulating human genes to identify and/or eliminate traits in our DNA. Most genes function by encoding synthesis of proteins and enzymes at the cellular level. The absence or defection of a gene can result in an array of different effects and defects. Being able to detect and/or manipulate those defects will greatly alter the course of allopathic medicine in the future.

Genetic testing can be performed to establish the identity of an individual or the relationship between individuals as in forensic medicine or paternity testing. It can be used to detect hereditary disorders in newborns, both prior to and after birth. The application of genetic testing to the specialty of oncology is increasingly more prevalent. Screening for oncogenes that indicate a predetermined risk for certain cancers is now a standard practice for many oncologists.

Rules & Exceptions

Obstetrics and Gynecology

abort, abortion
Transcribe this term as dictated (editing only as necessary for grammar and clarity). Although the AMA Manual of Style prefers the term *terminate* to *abort*, AAMT does not recommend making this editorial change if "abort" is dictated.

> DICTATED
> **abort**
>
> TRANSCRIBED
> **abort (not terminate)**

The abbreviations AB for abortion, SAB for spontaneous abortion (miscarriage), and TAB for therapeutic abortion are often used as well.

adnexa
Appendages or adjunct parts. The uterine adnexa consist of the ovaries, tubes, and ligaments. (The optical adnexa are the lids, lashes, brows, conjunctival sacs, lacrimal apparatus, and extrinsic muscles.) Adnexa is *always* plural, even when referring to only one side.

> **The adnexa are normal.**
> **Left adnexa are normal.**

APGAR questionnaire
Acronym from initial letters of adaptability, partnership, growth, affection, resolve, referring to a family assessment instrument. Use all capitals. Do not confuse with Apgar score.

Apgar score
Assessment of newborn's condition in which pulse, breathing, color, tone, and reflex irritability are each rated 0, 1, or 2, at one minute and five minutes after birth. Each set of ratings is totaled, and both totals are reported. Named after Virginia Apgar, MD. Do not con-

fuse with APGAR questionnaire for family assessment. Use initial capital only. Express ratings with arabic numerals. Write out the numbers related to minutes, in order to avoid confusion and to draw attention to the scores.

> **Apgars 7 and 9 at one and five minutes.**

GPA system

GPA is the abbreviation for *gravida, para, abortus*. Accompanied by arabic numerals, G, P, and A (or Ab) describe the patient's obstetric history. Use arabic numerals. Roman numerals are not appropriate.

G	gravida (number of pregnancies)
P	para (number of births of viable offspring)
A or Ab	abortus (abortions)

nulligravida	gravida 0	no pregnancies
primigravida	gravida 1, G1	1 pregnancy
secundigravida	gravida 2, G2	2 pregnancies
nullipara	para 0	no deliveries of viable offspring

Separate GPA sections by commas. Either the abbreviated or the spelled-out form may be used, whichever is dictated.

> **Obstetric history: G4, P3, A1.**
>
> *or*
>
> **Obstetric history: gravida 4, para 3, abortus 1.**

Pap smear

The brief form for Papanicolaou is Pap, which may be used if dictated. If the full word is dictated, transcribe in full.

NOTE: Be careful not to confuse *Pap* with *PAP*, which refers to *positive airway pressure* and relates to mechanical ventilation.

TPAL system System used to describe obstetric history of a patient.

> T   term infants
> P   premature infants
> A   abortions
> L   living children

Separate TPAL numbers by hyphens.

> **Obstetric history: 4-2-2-4**

TPAL numbers need not be spelled out unless dictated that way, for example:

> **Obstetric history: 4 term infants, 2 premature infants, 2 abortions, 4 living children.**

Sometimes, GPA terminology is combined with TPAL terminology.

> **The patient is gravida 3, 3-0-0-3.**
>
> *or*
>
> **The patient is gravida 3, para 3-0-0-3**
>
> *or*
>
> **The patient is G3, P3-0-0-3**
>
> *or*
>
> **The patient is gravida 3-0-0-3**

cesarean section Not *Cesarean*, *caesarean*, or *Caesarean*. Brief form is C-section, but do not use it unless it is dictated, and even then do not use it in the operative title section of operative reports or discharge summaries.

fundal height

Distance from symphysis pubis to dome (top) of uterus. Expressed in centimeters. After the 12th week of pregnancy, the number of centimeters should equal the number of weeks of pregnancy. If the measurement is larger, it may indicate large-for-dates fetus or multiple fetuses.

> **Fundal height is 28 cm.**

station

Term designating the location of the presenting fetal part in the birth canal. Expressed as -5 to +5, representing the number of centimeters below or above an imaginary plane through the ischial spines (station 0 is at the plane).

Genetics

chromosomal terms

There are 46 chromosomes in human cells, occurring in pairs and numbered 1 through 22, plus the sex chromosomes, an X and a Y in males and two X's in females. The non-sex chromosomes are also called autosomes.

group designations

Refer to chromosomes by number or by group.

chromosome	group
1-3	A
4, 5	B
6-12, X	C
13-15	D
16-18	E
19, 20	F
21, 22, Y	G

> **chromosome 16**
> **a chromosome in group E**
> **a group-E chromosome**

> **trisomy: an extra chromosome in any one of the autosomes or either sex chromosome**

trisomy D: an extra chromosome in a group-D chromosome, either the 13th, 14th, or 15th chromosome

trisomy 21: an extra 21st chromosome (Down syndrome)

A plus or minus in front of the chromosome number means there is either an extra chromosome or an absent chromosome within that pair.

trisomy 21 = female karyotype: 47,XX +21

The plus or minus following the chromosome number means that part of the chromosome is either extra or missing.

cri du chat syndrome = male karyotype: 46,X6 5p-

arms

Each chromosome has a short arm and a long arm. The short arm is designated by a p, the long arm by a q, immediately following the chromosome number (no space between). Each arm is divided into regions (from 1 to 4); place the region number immediately following the arm designation. Regions are divided into bands, again joined without a space. If a subdivision is identified, it follows a decimal point placed immediately after the band number.

20p	**20th chromosome, short arm**
20p1	**20th chromosome, short arm, region 1**
20p11	**20th chromosome, short arm, region 1, band 1**
20p11.23	**20th chromosome, short arm, region 1, band 1, subdivision 23**

A translocation occurs when a segment normally found in a certain arm of a chromosome appears in a different location; it may be written as a small t with the from and to sites in parentheses, e.g., t(14q21q), meaning from long arm of 14 to long arm of 21. A more complex designation such as t(2;6)(q34;p12) means from region 3 band 4 of the long arm of chromosome 2 to region 1 band 2 of the short arm of chromosome 6. The chromosome numbers appear in a separate set of parentheses from the arm, region, and band information.

A ring chromosome is one that has pieces missing from the end of each arm, and the two arms have joined at the ends.

bands

Use capital letters to refer to chromosome bands, which are elicited by special staining methods.

band	stain
C bands or C-banding	constitutive heterochromatin
G bands or G-banding	Giemsa
N bands or N-banding	nucleolar organizing region
Q bands or Q-banding	quinacrine
R bands or R-banding	reverse-Giemsa

karyotype

Describes an individual's chromosome complement: the number of chromosomes plus the sex chromosomes present in that individual. Place a comma (without spacing) between the chromosome number and the sex chromosome. Use a virgule to indicate more than one karyotype in an individual.

normal human karyotypes:	46,XX (female)
	46,XY (male)
some abnormal karyotypes:	47,XXY
	45,X0
	48,XXX
	45,X/46,XX

genes

Molecular units of heredity; their locations are called loci. A gene's main form and its locus have the same symbol, usually an abbreviation for the gene name or a quality of the gene. The symbol usually consists of 3 or 4 characters, all capitals, or all capitals and an arabic numeral, all on the line (no superscripts or subscripts). Do not use hyphens or spaces. Italics are used in formal publications, but regular type is preferred in medical transcription.

> **CF**   **cystic fibrosis**
> **G6PD** **glucose-6-phosphate dehydrogenase**
> **HPRT** **hypoxanthine phosphoriboxyltransferase**
> **PHP**   **panhypopituitarism**

Alleles are alternative forms of genes. To express their symbols, add an asterisk and the allele designation to the gene symbol. Italics are used in formal publications, but regular type is preferred in medical transcription.

> **HBB*6V**

biochemical constituents

The biochemical constituents of genetics include deoxyribonucleic acid, ribonucleic acid, and the amino acids.

deoxyribo-nucleic acid (DNA)

DNA includes the bases thymine (T), cytosine (C), adenine (A), and guanine (G). DNA contains the genetic code and is found in the chromosomes of humans and animals. DNA expressions and their abbreviations include:

> **complementary DNA**   **cDNA**
> **double-stranded DNA**   **dsDNA**
> **single-stranded DNA**   **ssDNA**

ribonucleic acid (RNA)

RNA includes the bases cytosine, adenine, guanine, and uracil (U). RNA is functionally associated with DNA. RNA expressions and their abbreviations include:

> **heterogeneous RNA**   **hnRNA**
> **messenger RNA**   **mRNA**
> **ribosomal RNA**   **rRNA**
> **small nuclear RNA**   **snRNA**
> **transfer RNA**   **tRNA**

amino acids of proteins

Write out in text. In tables, use three-letter or one-letter abbreviations.

phenylalanine	Phe	F
proline	Pro	P
tryptophan	rp	W

oncogenes

Viral genes in certain retroviruses. Express as three-letter lowercase terms derived from names of associated viruses. Italics are used in formal publications, but regular type is used in medical transcription.

abl
mos
sis
src

The prefix v- (virus) or c- (cellular or chromosomal counterpart) indicates the location of the oncogene. The c-prefixed oncogenes are also known as proto-oncogenes and may be alternatively expressed in all capitals, without the prefix. Italics are used in formal publications, but regular type is preferred in medical transcription. Note: The prefix is never italicized.

human leukocyte antigen (HLA)

Test that detects genetic markers on white blood cells. Abbreviation: HLA. Express with capital-lowercase combinations and hyphens. Check appropriate references for guidance.

HLA-DR5   associated with Hashimoto thyroiditis
B8, Dw3   associated with Graves disease

major histocompatibility complex, class I antigens

HLA-D
HLA-DR

major histocompatibility complex, class II antigens

HLA-B27
HLA-DRw10

examples of antigenic specificities of major HLA loci

HLA-A
HLA-B
HLA-C
HLA-D

The Final Word

The information provided in this chapter related to genetics is very complex and encountered infrequently in mainstream dictation. However, you will likely continue to hear more references to genetics and genomic research through your career. Probably more than any medical transcriptionists who came before you, you will represent the generation of MTs whose work is greatly impacted by research in the genomic discipline. It is best to be prepared for that reality now. The standards you have covered in the obstetrics and gynecology section, however, are very commonplace, and you should be prepared to encounter those wherever you go in the industry.

Test Your Knowledge

Correct the errors in each of the sentences below.

---

1. She is gravida-2, para-1, ab-2, and her last menstrual period was in 1958.

2. PREOPERATIVE DIAGNOSIS: Previous Cesarean section.

3. A live female newborn, Apgars 99 at 1 and 5 minutes, weight 4310 gm, was delivered.

4. On examination, the adnexae were normal.

5. The patient was taken back to the delivery room after 3-1/4 hours of pushing and 3+ station.

6. The remaining 48 cells were of normal female karyotype (46-XX).

7. She was 80% effaced with cervix dilated to 4 cm, and the fetus was noted to be at minus 2 station.

8. This is a G3/P2-1-0-3 female who presents today with vaginal bleeding.

9. She delivered a female weighing 8 lb 5 oz and sustained a fourth degree laceration.

10. Obstetrical history: Gravida 4, para 3-0-1-4.

APPLICATION TEST
Take the application test for this chapter on your CD-ROM. Access the section for
Chapter 16: "**Obstetrics, Gynecology & Genetics.**"

Test Your Knowledge

Answers

1.	She is gravida 2, para 1, Ab 2, and her last menstrual period was in 1958.
2.	PREOPERATIVE DIAGNOSIS: Previous cesarean section.
3.	A live female newborn, Apgars 9 and 9 at one and five minutes, weight 4310 g, was delivered.
4.	On examination, the adnexa were normal.
5.	The patient was taken back to the delivery room after 3-1/4 hours of pushing and +3 station.
6.	The remaining 48 cells were of normal female karyotype (46,XX).
7.	She was 80% effaced with cervix dilated to 4 cm, and the fetus was noted to be at -2 station.
8.	This is a G3, P2-1-0-3 female who presents today with vaginal bleeding.
9.	She delivered a female weighing 8 pounds 5 ounces and sustained a fourth-degree laceration.
10.	Obstetrical history: Gravida 4, para 3-0-1-3.

Note: A gravida 4 female who has had 1 abortion could not have a para history that reflects 4 living children. Edit appropriately or flag to the dictator's attention.

Orthopedics/ Neurology & Surgery

The transcription of operative reports has been deemed by many an MT to be among the most challenging of clinical documentation work types. In the acute care setting, operative reports make up a significant portion of the daily load of transcription for an MT in medical records. Of these, in any major facility, orthopedic and neurologic procedures comprise a substantial section of those operative reports.

These specialties provide a diverse, rich language that is unique and fascinating. Where else will you encounter such unusual phrases and acronyms as *FOOSH (fell on outstretched hand), catch and clunk test, boutonnière deformity, breakdancer's thumb, Stookey reflex, microknurling,* and *matricectomy*? With myriad tests associated with reflex, sensation, mobility, gait, and neurological function, the eponyms alone can keep an MT running to the reference books. In addition, no other specialty can boast such a surprising repertoire of unique surgical instruments and materials (*rasps, rongeurs, curettes, saws, cement, plates, pins, screws, wires, reamers, perforators, retractors,* etc.). You will find that operative reports in orthopedics sound more like an episode of *This Old House* than they do a clinical procedure! Orthopedic surgery could be described as "applied anatomical carpentry," as the methods and techniques used to reinforce and correct the deformities and conditions of the skeleton are very similar to those applied to any other *structure.*

This chapter will orient you to the standards of style specific to these areas. Ideally, this section should be studied in conjunction with learning the anatomy, physiology, disease processes, etc., related to these complex specialties. Attempting to work through this chapter without a fundamental understanding of the anatomy and physiology and disease processes related to these specialties could prove confusing and difficult. This chapter should also be coordinated with transcription application in this area so that the standards covered here can be reinforced through hands-on practice.

Going Deeper

Given the specific challenges of transcribing orthopedic and neurologic surgery, this chapter will provide not only the standards of style that relate to these specialties, but also the standards found in the *Book of Style* that are specific to general surgical terminology and instrumentation. There are not enough standards in the *Book of Style* that relate specifically to surgery to warrant a chapter of their own, so they are included here in conjunction with one of the most challenging surgical specialties. Therefore, some of these standards may seem out of context with orthopedics or neurology, but they are provided here as an orientation to *surgery* in general.

Rules & Exceptions

anatomic terms

Features. Do not capitalize the names of anatomic features (except the eponyms associated with them).

> **os frontale**
> **zygomatic bone**
> **ligament of Treitz**

Posture-based terms:

anterior	nearer the front
posterior	nearer the rear
superior	nearer the top
inferior	nearer the bottom

Region-based terms:

cranial, cephalic	nearer the head
caudal	nearer the tail or lower end
dorsal	nearer the back
ventral	nearer the belly side or anterior surface

Directional and positional terms. Form directional adverbs by replacing the adjectival suffix (-al, -or, -ic) with the suffix -ad, meaning -*ward*. Use these forms in the same type of constructions in which -*ward* forms are used.

caudad
cephalad
craniad
laterad
orad
superiad
ventrad

Do not substitute the -*ad* form when the adjective itself or the -*ly* adverb has been used correctly.

**It extends caudally from...
the anterior incision**

Use a combining vowel to join directional and positional adjectives.

mediolateral

Latin and English names. It is common practice to mix the English and Latin names of anatomic parts, e.g., using English for the noun and Latin for the adjectives. These may be transcribed as dictated or edited to either their English or Latin forms.

> **latissimus dorsi muscle**
> **peroneus profundus nerve**
> **palpebrales arteries**

angles

Orthopedics. In expressing angles, write out degrees or use degree sign (°).

> **The patient was able to straight leg raise to 40 degrees.**
>
> *or* **...to 40°.**

Imaging studies. Use the degree sign (°) in imaging studies.

> **Positioning the patient's head at a 90° angle allowed for efficient acquisition of data over a 180° arc.**
> **Coronary cineangiography was done to LAO 60°, RAO 30°.**

If the symbol is not available, spell out degree or degrees.

> **a 90-degree angle...a 180-degree arc**
> **30-degree LAO, 30-degree cranial**

body cavities

Body spaces containing internal organs.

cavity	organs
cranial	brain
thoracic	esophagus, trachea, thymus gland, aorta, lungs, heart
abdominal	gallbladder, liver, spleen, pancreas, stomach, small intestine, large intestine

pelvic	urinary bladder, urethra, ureters (in female: uterus and vagina, as well)
spinal	nerves of spinal cord

body parts

Phrases such as left heart and right chest are frequently dictated when what is meant is left side of heart, right side of chest. These phrases may be transcribed as dictated unless their usage would confuse or amuse rather than communicate.

left heart catheterization
right chest abscess
left neck incision

cranial nerves

Use arabic or roman numerals for cranial nerve designations. Be consistent. (Employer or client will often indicate preference.)

cranial nerve 12	cranial nerve XII
cranial nerves 2-12	cranial nerves II-XII

Ordinals should be expressed using arabic numerals or may be spelled out in full.

12th cranial nerve

or

twelfth cranial nerve

English names are preferred to Latin, but transcribe Latin forms if they are dictated.

number	English name	Latin name
1 or I	olfactory	olfactorius
2 or II	optic	opticus
3 or III	oculomotor	oculomotorius
4 or IV	trochlear	trochlearis
5 or V	trigeminal	trigeminus

6 or VI	abducens	abducens
7 or VII	facial	facialis
8 or VIII	vestibulocochlear	vestibulocochlearis
9 or IX	glossopharyngeal	glossopharyngeus
10 or X	vagus	vagus
11 or XI	accessory	accessorius
12 or XII	hypoglossal	hypoglossus

crepitance, crepitation crepitus

Crepitus, *crepitation*, and *crepitance* are all synonymous. The adjectival form is crepitant ("crepitants" is not a word). Although crepitance is not found in dictionaries, its frequent usage has made it acceptable.

Electro-encephalographic terms

EEG: Abbreviation for electroencephalogram, electroencephalography, and electroencephalograph.

Symbols for electrodes. Use capital letters to refer to anatomic areas. Use subscript lowercase letters to refer to relative electrode positions. Use subscript odd numbers to refer to electrodes placed on the left. Subscript even numbers refer to those on the right; subscript z refers to midline (zero) electrodes. If subscripts are not available, place the lowercase letters, numbers, and z on the line, adjacent to the capital letter and to each other, or spell out the terms.

A1, A2	A_1, A_2	earlobe electrodes
Cz, C3, C4	C_z, C_3, C_4	central electrodes
F7, F8	F_7, F_8	anterior temporal electrodes
Fpz, Fp1, Fp2	F_{pz}, F_{p1}, F_{p2}	frontal pole; prefrontal electrodes
Fz, F3, F4	F_z, F_3, F_4	frontal electrodes
Oz, O1, O2	O_z, O_1, O_2	occipital electrodes
Pg1, Pg2	P_{g1}, P_{g2}	nasopharyngeal electrodes
Pz, P3, P4	P_z, P_3, P_4	parietal electrodes
T3, T4	T_3, T_4	midtemporal electrodes
T5, T6	T_5, T_6	posterior temporal electrodes

Frequency. Express in cycles per second (c/s or cps) or hertz (Hz).

> **16 c/s *or* 16 cps *or* 16 Hz**

Some terms commonly used in EEG reports:

> **alert, drowsy, and sleeping states**
> **alpha range**
> **alpha rhythm**
> **alpha waves**
> **amplitude**
> **artifact**
> **background rhythm**
> **beta rhythms**
> **bisynchronous**
> **central sleep spindles**
> **cycles per second (c/s, cps)**
> **delta brush**
> **delta spikes**
> **delta waves**
> **frontal sharp transient**
> **hyperventilation**
> **lambda rhythm**
> **lateralizing focus**
> **mu pattern**
> **occipital driving**
> **paroxysmal, paroxysms**
> **photic stimulation**
> **rhythmic activity**
> **sharp elements**
> **sharp waves**
> **sleep spindles**
> **slow transients**
> **slow waves**
> **spike and dome complex**
> **spike and wave pattern**
> **spikes**
> **spindles**
> **Standard International lead placements**
> **symmetrical activity**
> **synchronous**

> **theta activity**
> **theta frequency**
> **21-channel recording**
> **vertex waves**
> **voltage**
> **wave bursts**

fingerbreadth   Plural form is *fingerbreadths* not *fingersbreadth*.

fluctuance,   *Fluctuation* and *fluctuance* are synonymous.
fluctuation
NOTE: *Fluctuants* is not a word.

> **The adjectival form is fluctuant.**

Fluctuance was not found in dictionaries until 2000 when it was added to the 27th edition of *Stedman's Medical Dictionary* as a secondary spelling for *fluctuation*.

fracture-   Use a hyphen, as indicated.
dislocation

French scale   Sizing system for catheters, sounds, and other tubular instruments. Each unit is approximately 0.33 mm in diameter. Precede by # or *No.* if the word "number" is dictated. Capitalize *French*.

> **5-French catheter**
> **#5-French catheter**
> **catheter, size 5 French**

Keep in mind that French is linked to diameter size and is not the eponymic name of an instrument. Thus, it is a 15-French catheter, not a French catheter, size 15.

magnification   **X**. Magnification is generally expressed with a capital X (although a lowercase x is acceptable) placed before the size of magnification, without a space.

> **X30 magnification**

Loupe magnification. A loupe is a magnifying lens. *Loop* is not an acceptable alternative.

meridians

Imaginary location lines that circle a globular structure, such as the eye, at right angles to its equator and touching both poles. Measured in units of 0 degrees to 180 degrees.

> **The eye was entered at the 160-degree meridian.**

In acupuncture, meridians connect different anatomic sites.

operate, operate on

A surgeon operates on a patient, and a patient is operated on. Add *on* even if not dictated.

> DICTATED
> **The patient was operated without incident.**
>
> TRANSCRIBED
> **The patient was operated on without incident.**

pins, screws, wires

Orthopedic pins, screws, and wires are generally measured in portions of an inch.

> DICTATED
> **a three thirty two Steinmann pin**
>
> TRANSCRIBED
> **a 3/32-inch Steinmann pin**

Kirschner wires are measured in portions of an inch but written using decimals.

> DICTATED
> **a four five K wire and a six two K wire**
>
> TRANSCRIBED
> **a 0.045 K-wire and a 0.062 K-wire**

plane   An imaginary flat surface.

Planes of the body and its structures include those listed below. Check appropriate references (anatomy books and medical dictionaries) for additional planes.

frontal   A vertical plane dividing the body or structure into anterior and posterior portions. Also known as coronal plane.

sagittal   Lengthwise vertical plane dividing the body or structure into right and left portions; midsagittal plane divides the body into right and left halves. Also known as median plane.

transverse   Plane running across the body parallel to the ground, dividing the body or structure into upper and lower portions. Also known as horizontal or axial plane.

plain film   Indicates that the x-ray was done without contrast.
x-rays   Not a CT scan, just a plain x-ray. Not *plane*.

> **Plain film of the abdomen was negative.**

post, post-   Post is a prefix that can sometimes stand on its own as a word (meaning after); it can also serve as an inseparable prefix.

> **The patient should follow up 1 week post discharge.**
> **She is 3 weeks status post breast biopsy.**
> **Her postoperative pain has been minimal.**

In the following example, the word post is used as part of a hyphenated compound modifier.

> **post-mastectomy scar**

reflexes   Graded 0 to 4.

Express as an arabic numeral followed (or preceded) by a plus sign (except 0, which stands alone). Lowercase the word *grade*.

grade	meaning
0	absent
+1 *or* 1+	decreased
+2 *or* 2+	normal
+3 *or* 3+	hyperactive
+4 *or* 4+	clonus

DICTATED
grade 2 to 3 plus over 4

TRANSCRIBED
grade 2+/4 to 3+/4

Do not use plus signs without the numeral, i.e., do not use +, ++, +++, ++++.

Knee reflexes were grade 3+/4.
not **...grade +++/4.**

subcu   Abbreviated form for subcutaneous or subcuticular. When *subcu* is dictated and you are unsure which term is intended, spell *subcu* or *subcut*. Do not use the abbreviation *sub q* because the *q* can be mistaken for a medication dosage.

DICTATED
The wound was closed with running subcu stitches of 5-0 Prolene.

TRANSCRIBED
The wound was closed with running subcu stitches of 5-0 Prolene.

super-, supra-   *Super-* means more than, above, superior, or in the upper part of the term to which it is joined.

supernumerary (more than the usual number)
superolateral (in the upper part of the lateral aspect)

Supra- means in a position above the part of the term to which it is joined.

> **supraclavicular**
> **supraglottic**
> **supraorbital**
> **suprapubic**
> **supraventricular**

Although the meanings of *super-* and *supra-* sometimes overlap, the two are not generally interchangeable. Both prefixes are generally joined directly to the following term without a hyphen, but the usual exceptions apply. Check dictionaries and other appropriate references for guidance as to the correct prefix and how it is joined.

suture sizes

USP system. The United States Pharmacopeia system sizes, among other things, steel sutures and sutures of other materials. The sizes range from 11-0 (smallest) to 7 (largest). Thus, a size 7 suture is different from and larger than a size 7-0 suture. Use 0 or 1-0 for single-aught suture; use the "digit hyphen zero" style to express sizes 2-0 through 11-0. Express sizes 1 through 7 with whole numbers. Place the symbol # before the size if *number* is dictated.

> **1-0 nylon or 0 nylon**
> **2-0 nylon not 00 nylon**
> **4-0 Vicryl not 0000 Vicryl**
> **#7 cotton not 0000000 cotton**

> DICTATED
> **3 and 4 oh silk**
>
> TRANSCRIBED
> **3-0 and 4-0 silk**

Brown and Sharp gauge (B&S gauge): System for sizing stainless steel sutures. Use whole arabic numerals ranging from 40 (smallest) to 20 (largest). Thus, a size 30 suture is smaller than a size 25.

Veress needle   The correct spelling is *Veress*, although many continue to use the incorrect spelling with two *r's* and one *s*. In the introduction dated July 1992 to *Vera Pyle's Current Medical Terminology*, the author remarks on an article written by a Dr. Veress, the developer of the Veress needle, thus confirming the spelling.

vertebra   Expressed by a capital C, T, L, or S to indicate the region (cervical, thoracic, lumbar, or sacral), followed by an arabic numeral placed on the line (do not subscript or superscript). D for dorsal is sometimes substituted for T (thoracic). Do not use a hyphen between the letter and the number of a specific vertebra. Do not subscript or superscript the numerals. Plural: vertebrae.

> **S1 *not* S-1**
> **T2 *or* D2**

It is preferable to repeat the letter before each numbered vertebra in a list.

> **The lesion involves C4, C5, and C6.**
> ***not* ...C4, 5, and 6.**
> ***and not* ...C4, 5, 6.**

Intervertebral disk space. Use a hyphen to express the space between two vertebrae (the intervertebral space). It is not necessary to repeat the same letter before the second vertebra, but it may be transcribed if dictated.

> **C1-2 *or* C1-C2**
> **L5-S1**

The Final Word

Transcribing operative reports can often feel like you are right there in the procedure room with the physician. In fact, in the early days of patient care documentation, medical secretaries often sat in a corner of the operating room, taking shorthand notes from the physician, who dictated throughout the procedure. Those notes were later transcribed on a manual typewriter for inclusion in the patient's record. While those days are long behind us, operative reports are still a critical part of the care record, and most MTs find them to be among the most interesting reports they are tasked with transcribing. New MTs, however, can find complex procedures to be challenging and frustrating. In specialties like Orthopedics and Neurology, the anatomical terms, surgical equipment references, and procedural flow can be particularly complex. The investment of time, however, in acclimating to operative report transcription can pay big dividends down the road. Once learned, operative notes lend themselves well to word expanders and templates, given their highly repetitive and predictable nature, particularly with common procedures.

Test Your Knowledge

Correct the errors in each of the sentences below.

---

1. Deep tendon reflexes were bilaterally symmetrical, with upper extremities 1-2+/2 and lower extremities 2+/2.

2. The right hip showed slightly better range of motion with flexion of approximately 80 degrees, abduction of 10-15 degrees, and 15 degree fixed external rotation.

3. There was gross instability of the left medio-collateral ligament and anterior cruciate ligament with a positive McMurray maneuver to suggest an O'Donoghue's Triad.

4. There was no evidence of fracture on plane films.

5. Skin was closed with running 4.0 Ethilon.

6. The osteotomy site was fixed via the use of a 45 Kirschner wire.

7. The patient was catheterized with a No. 16 french Foley catheter.

8. DIAGNOSIS: Subluxation, L-5/S-1.

9. There was an area of tenderness 3 fingersbreadth below the umbilicus.

10. She is now 6 weeks postsurgery and is here for followup.

Test Your Knowledge

Answers

1. Deep tendon reflexes were bilaterally symmetrical, with upper extremities 1+/2 to 2+/2 and lower extremities 2+/2.

2. The right hip showed slightly better range of motion with flexion of approximately 80 degrees, abduction of 10-15 degrees, and 15-degree fixed external rotation.

3. There was gross instability of the left medial collateral ligament and anterior cruciate ligament with a positive McMurray maneuver to suggest an O'Donoghue triad.

4. There was no evidence of fracture on plain films.

5. Skin was closed with running 4-0 Ethilon.

6. The osteotomy site was fixed via the use of a 0.045 Kirschner wire.

7. The patient was catheterized with a No. 16-French Foley catheter. *or* The patient was catheterized with a #16-French Foley catheter.

8. DIAGNOSIS: Subluxation, L5-S1.

9. There was an area of tenderness 3 fingerbreadths below the umbilicus.

10. She is now 6 weeks post surgery and is here for followup.

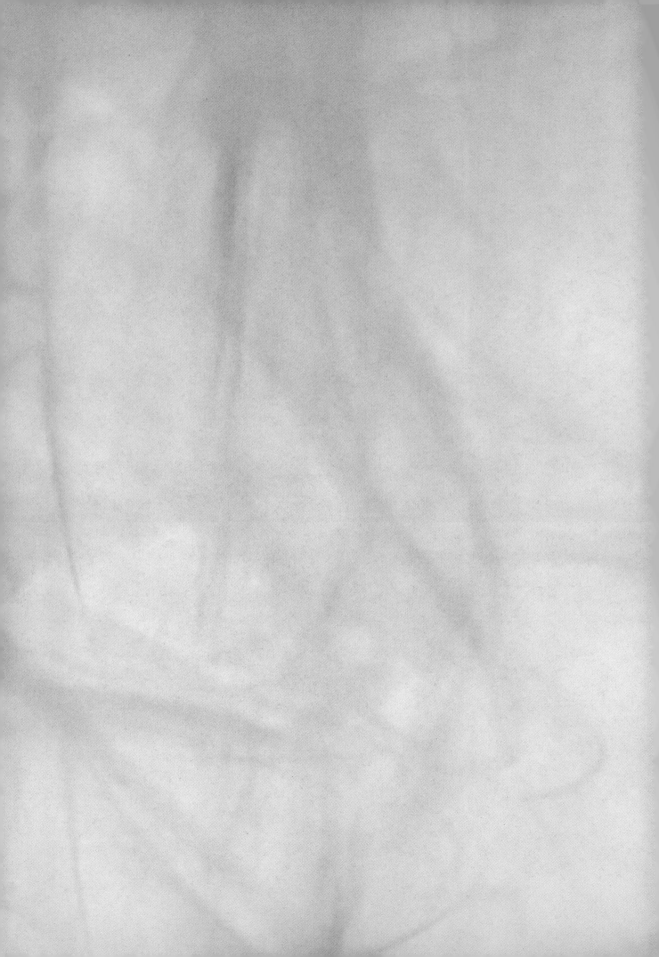

Other Standards

Foreign Terms and Derivations

The current lexicography of medical language is vast and complex. This living and constantly evolving language has been profoundly influenced over time by a diverse number of cultural and linguistic sources, many of which are still evident in the language today. While certainly the English medical terms with which we are familiar can be etymologically traced to earlier language forms, there are quite a few foreign terms that remain unaltered in circular usage today.

Going Deeper

The influence of foreign language is evident throughout medical terminology. Most anatomical terms are either derived from the Latin or Greek (*abdomen* from *abdominis*) or still referred to by their Latin or Greek names (*rectus abdominis, flexor digitorum profundus,* etc.). Medical language is also peppered with other terms of international origin, such as French (*torsade de pointes, curettage, cerclage,* etc.) and German (*blitz, ersatz, mittelschmerz,* etc.). When encountered in dictation, they should be transcribed as dictated, with the exception that providers are not always accurate in the dictation of singular and plural forms of Latin and Greek terms. This chapter will provide insight into the standards as they relate to foreign terms, but pay particular attention to the rules for singular and plural forms of these terms. As a medical transcriptionist, you will be expected to recognize the context of these terms and determine if the singular or plural form is appropriate, regardless of how the term may be dictated.

Rules & Exceptions

abbreviations

e.g., et al., etc., i.e., viz. These Latin abbreviations are commonly used in English communications and need not be translated, although the medical transcriptionist should understand their meaning before using them. The use of periods within or at the end of these Latin abbreviations remains the preferred style, although it is also acceptable to drop the periods.

abbreviation	Latin	English
e.g. *or* eg	exempli gratia	for example
et al. *or* et al	et alii	and others
etc. *or* etc	et cetera	and so forth
i.e. *or* ie	id est	that is
viz. *or* viz	videlicet	that is, namely

Use a comma before and after the abbreviation (or its English equivalent).

Her symptoms come on with exertion, e.g., when climbing stairs or running.
Her symptoms come on with exertion, for example, when climbing stairs or running.
She continued to be uncooperative, i.e., she refused all treatment.
She continued to be uncooperative, that is, she refused all treatment.

Drug-related abbreviations. Use lowercase abbreviations with periods for Latin abbreviations that are related to doses and dosages. Do not use abbreviations found on the "Dangerous Abbreviations" list from the Institute for Safe Medication Practices. Avoid using all capitals because they emphasize the abbreviation rather than the drug name. Avoid lowercase abbreviations without periods because some may be misread as words. Do not translate.

abbreviation	Latin phrase	English translation
a.c.	ante cibum	before food
b.i.d.	bis in die	twice a day
gtt.	guttae	drops (better to spell out *drops*)
n.p.o.	nil per os	nothing by mouth
n.r.	non repetatur	do not repeat
p.c.	post cibum	after food
p.o.	per os	by mouth
p.r.n.	pro re nata	as needed
q.4 h.	quaque 4 hora	every 4 hours
q.h.	quaque hora	every hour
q.i.d.	quater in die	4 times a day
t.i.d.	ter in die	3 times a day
u.d.	ut dictum	as directed

NOTE: We have inserted a space after the numeral *4* in *q.4 h.* on the advice of the ISMP so that the number is more easily and clearly read.

Invalid Latin abbreviations such as *q.a.m.* (every morning) and mixed Latin and English abbreviations such as *q.4 hours* (every 4 hours) have become commonplace. However, as with all abbreviations, avoid those that are obscure (like *a.c.b.* for before breakfast) or dangerous. For example, *b.i.w.* is both obscure and dangerous. It is intended to mean twice weekly but it could be mistaken for twice daily, resulting in a dosage frequency seven times that intended.

adnexa

Appendages or adjunct parts. The uterine adnexa consist of the ovaries, tubes, and ligaments. The optical adnexa are the lids, lashes, brows, conjunctival sacs, lacrimal apparatus, and extrinsic muscles. Adnexa is always plural, even when referring to only one side.

> **The adnexa are normal.**
> **Left adnexa are normal.**
> **The ocular adnexa are normal on the right.**

data, datum

Data, the plural form of *datum*, usually takes a plural verb, but its use as a collective noun taking a singular verb is becoming widely accepted. The singular form, datum, is seldom used.

> **The data were collected over a period of several years.**
> **The data demonstrates conclusive evidence that . . .**
> **The research data were checked, datum by datum.**

foreign terms   Do not italicize foreign abbreviations, words, and phrases used in medical reports. Capitalize, punctuate, and space according to the standards of the language of origin. Omit accent marks except in proper names or where current usage retains them.

> **cul-de-sac**
> **en masse**
> **facade**
> **i.e.**
> **in vivo**
> **naive**
> **peau d'orange**

Do not translate foreign words or abbreviations unless the originator translates them.

**genus and
species names**   A genus includes species whose broad features are alike in organization but different in detail.

A species is a group of individuals that can interbreed and produce fertile offspring. A species name is usually preceded by its genus name.

Capitalization. Always capitalize genus names and their abbreviated forms when they are accompanied by a species name. Always lowercase species names.

> **Haemophilus influenzae**
> **Escherichia coli**
> **Staphylococcus aureus**

Lowercase genus names used in plural and adjectival forms and when used in the vernacular, for example, when they stand alone (without a species name).

> **staphylococcus**
> **group B streptococcus**
> **staphylococci**
> **staphylococcal infection**
> **staph infection**
> **strep throat**

-osis, -iasis. The suffixes *-osis* and *-iasis* indicate disease caused by a particular class of infectious agents or types of infection. Lowercase terms formed with these suffixes.

Greek letters   Spell out the English translation when the word stands alone. Do not capitalize English translations. Use the Greek letter or spell it out when it is part of an extended term, according to the preferred form; consult appropriate references for guidance.

> **alpha** α
> **beta** β
> **gamma** γ

In extended terms, use of a hyphen after the Greek letter is optional, but the hyphen is not used after the English translation.

> **β-globulin or B globulin**
> **beta globulin**

plurals   **Medical terms derived from Latin or Greek.** General rules follow. Consult appropriate medical dictionaries for additional guidance.

Words ending in *-en*

Change text ending to *-ina*.

> **foramen**   **foramina**

Words ending in *-a*

Add *-e*.

conjunctiva	conjunctivae

Words ending in *-us*

Change ending to *-i*.

meniscus	menisci
embolus	emboli

EXCEPTIONS

meatus	meatus
processus	processus

Words ending in *-on*

Change ending to *-a*.

ganglion	ganglia

Words ending in *-is*

Change ending to *-es*.

diagnosis	diagnoses

EXCEPTIONS

arthritis	arthritides
epididymis	epididymides

Words ending in *-um*

Change ending to *-a*.

diverticulum	diverticula

The plural forms of Latin terms that consist of a noun-adjective combination are often difficult to determine. (In Latin, the adjective must agree in number, gender, and case with the noun it modifies.) In the following list we show such terms in their singular and plural forms; they are all in the nominative case.

singular	plural
processus vaginalis	processus vaginales
chorda tendinea	chordae tendineae
verruca vulgaris	verrucae vulgares
nucleus pulposus	nuclei pulposi
pars interarticularis	partes interarticulares
placenta previa	placentae previae
musculus trapezius	musculi trapezii

Sometimes the genitive case (used in Latin to show possession) is misread as a plural, causing confusion. The following terms consist, for the most part, of a noun in the nominative case plus a noun in the genitive case.

Latin term	English translation
abruptio placentae	rupture of the placenta
bulbus urethrae	bulb of the urethra, bulbous urethra
cervix uteri	neck of uterus, uterine cervix
chondromalacia patellae	chondromalacia of the patella
corpus uteri	body of uterus, uterine corpus
os calcis	bone(s) of the heel(s); (plural: ossa calcium)
os coxae	bone(s) of the hip(s); (plural: ossa coxae)
pars uterina placentae	part of the placenta derived from uterine tissue
pruritus vulvae	itching of the vulva
muscularis mucosa	muscular (layer) of mucosa
lamina muscularis mucosae	muscular (layer) of mucosa

The Final Word

Medical language is diverse and complex, arising from adoption and usage of terms from a variety of sources. The migration and merging of disparate societies, the evolution of language over thousands of years, and the historic collaborative effort of scientists and physicians from around the world have yielded a compendium of clinical language that is as much a literary melting pot as the United States is a cultural one. The lifelong student of this language will never be bored, for it is as rich as it is vast. The best MTs develop a love affair with medical language over time, and evolve a working clinical vocabulary that greatly aids the application of the MT skill set in the workplace. We become collectors of dictionaries and etymology texts that feed our curiosity and fascination with the origin and meaning of medical words. Students who do not enter the profession with an inherent love of words may struggle to acclimate to this language-intense profession and would do well to spend extra time in fundamental terminology to create that foundation on which to build.

Test Your Knowledge

I. For each of the singular forms below, provide the plural form.

1. criterion _____

2. arthritis _____

3. phenomenon _____

4. meniscus _____

5. urethra _____

6. nucleus pulposus _____

7. uterus _____

8. placenta previa _____

9. diagnosis _____

10. foramen _____

II. For each of the plural forms below, provide the singular form.

11. diverticula _____

12. epididymides _____

13. stamina _____

14. adnexa _____

15. biceps _____

16. conjunctivae _____

17. cerebra _____

18. verrucae vulgares _____

19. musculi trapezii _____

20. ganglia _____

III. **Correct the errors in each of the sentences below.**

1. X-rays of the cervical spine showed cervical spondylosis with encroachment on the neural foramen of C5 and C6.

2. The breasts contained no masses and axilla are free of nodes.

3. She states she drinks only occasionally, e.g. a beer or two on the weekend or a glass of wine with dinner.

4. The patient was given PO Tylenol and discharged to take the same at home PRN.

5. Cultures were positive for Staph Aureus and she will be treated empirically for that.

6. Examination of the adnexa are normal.

7. DIAGNOSIS: Patent ductus arteriosis.

8. The transverse abdominal, internal oblique, and external oblique muscle and fascia were then approximated using a 3-0 running Vicryl suture.

9. HEENT: Sclera anicteric. Conjunctiva clear.

10. Examination of the transverse colon revealed multiple inflamed diverticuli.

Test Your Knowledge

Answers

I.		II.	
1.	criteria	**11.**	diverticulum
2.	arthritides	**12.**	epididymis
3.	phenomena	**13.**	stamen
4.	menisci	**14.**	adnexa
5.	urethrae	**15.**	biceps
6.	nuclei polposi	**16.**	conjunctiva
7.	uteri	**17.**	cerebrum
8.	placentae previae	**18.**	verruca vulgaris
9.	diagnoses	**19.**	musculus trapezius
10.	foramina	**20.**	ganglion

III.

1. X-rays of the cervical spine showed cervical spondylosis with encroachment on the neural foramina of C5 and C6.

2. The breasts contained no masses and axillae are free of nodes.

3. She states she drinks only occasionally, e.g., a beer or two on the weekend or a glass of wine with dinner.

4. The patient was given p.o. Tylenol and discharged to take the same at home p.r.n.

5. Cultures were positive for Staphylococcus aureus and she will be treated empirically for that.

6. Examination of the adnexa is normal.

7. DIAGNOSIS: Patent ductus arteriosus.

8. The transverse abdominal, internal oblique, and external oblique muscles and fasciae were then approximated using a 3-0 running Vicryl suture.

9. HEENT: Sclerae anicteric. Conjunctivae clear.

10. Examination of the transverse colon revealed multiple inflamed diverticula.

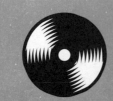

APPLICATION TEST
Take the application test for this chapter on your CD-ROM.
Access the section for
Chapter 18: "Foreign Terms and Derivations."

The Medical Record: Types and Formats

While all documentation recorded of a patient's care is considered a legal part of the medical record, medical transcriptionists are responsible primarily for the narrative portions of the patient record that detail the diagnostic decision-making process surrounding a patient's care. In a private practice or clinical setting, this includes the history and physical report or letter generated on the patient's first visit to the office, followup visit notes, letters to referring physicians and third parties, and documentation of phone correspondence with the patient. In the acute care setting, however, this involves what is typically referred to as the "Basic Four," i.e., admitting history and physical reports, consultations, operative reports, and discharge summaries. On a specialty basis, of course, transcription can cover radiology, special procedure, pathology, and diagnostic testing reports.

This chapter focuses on those standards of style related to document formatting, and provides definitions for the major document types. The standards outlined here are based on research of industry trends and practices, as well as those standards for formatting that are outlined by ASTM (American Society of Testing and Materials), the organization that establishes and promotes standards for all industries, including transcription.

Going Deeper

As a student, you are probably looking to this chapter as a guide for document formatting. Most students have a strong desire for concrete, black-and-white instructions for "how" to transcribe any given material. It will be important to understand in this chapter, probably more than any other, that these are *guidelines* for document formatting, and that adoption of formatting standards varies greatly from one facility to the next. The standards related to *correspondence*, for example are AAMT's recommendations for formatting letters, emails, etc., but you should be prepared for flexibility where document formats are concerned, as you may work for one provider who has strong preferences about style and format that may not necessarily concur with those outlined here. Always remember it is *clarity of communication* that guides standards in medical transcription, and in those instances where clarity is not compromised by a facility's preference for format, the MT should not be overly concerned about the departure from those standards outlined here.

Rules & Exceptions

autopsy report	Report prepared by a pathologist or medical examiner to document findings on examination of a cadaver. Typical content topics include medical history, course of treatment, external and internal examinations, evidence of injury, macroscopic and microscopic examinations, gross findings (systems and organs), special dissections, pathologic diagnosis, and cause of death.
character spacing	When using a proportional-spaced font it is customary to mark the end of a sentence with a single space; however, double-spacing is still widely used, especially with non-proportional fonts, such as Courier. The choice is usually determined by departmental or company policy.

Use either a single character space or two spaces (but be consistent in your usage) after

- the end of a sentence, whether it ends in a period, question mark, exclamation point, quotation mark, parenthesis, bracket, or brace

- a colon used as a punctuation mark within a sentence

Use a single character space after

- each word or symbol (unless the next character is a punctuation mark)
- a comma
- a semicolon
- a period at the end of an abbreviation

Use a single character space before

- an opening quotation mark
- an opening parenthesis
- an opening bracket or brace

Do not use a character space before or after

- an apostrophe (except when the apostrophe ends the term, as in the plural possessive patients', in which case a space or another punctuation mark follows the apostrophe)
- a colon in expressions of time or clock or equator positions, e.g., 1:30
- a colon in expressions of ratios and dilutions, e.g., 1:100,000
- a comma in numeric expressions, e.g., 12,034
- a decimal point in numeric expressions (except in those rare instances when a unit less than 1 does not call for a zero to be placed before the decimal, e.g., .22-caliber rifle, in which instances a space precedes the decimal point but does not follow it)
- a decimal point in monetary expressions, e.g., $1.50
- a hyphen, e.g., 3-0 suture material
- a dash, e.g.: Episodes of dyspnea—usually without pain—occur on slight exertion.
- a virgule, e.g., 2/6 heart murmur
- a period within an abbreviation, e.g., q.i.d.
- an ampersand in abbreviations such as T&A, D&C

Do not use a character space after

- an opening quotation mark
- an opening parenthesis, bracket, or brace
- a word followed by a punctuation mark

Do not use a character space before

- a punctuation mark (except an opening parenthesis, bracket, brace, or quotation mark)

consultation report A consultation includes examination, review, and assessment of a patient by a healthcare provider other than the attending physician. The report generated is called a consultation report. The consulting specialist directs the report to the physician requesting the consultation, usually the attending physician. Content usually includes patient examination, review, and assessment. It may be prepared in letter or report format.

correspondence Patient reports often are written in the form of a letter to a referring or consulting physician. The fonts, styles, and margins chosen for use in letters may differ from those used in other medical reports; each department (or client) will develop its own policies.

Letter formats and styles. Margins for letters are often determined by the letterhead used. It is not uncommon in long letters that additional pages conform to different margins, depending on the paper used. Be sure to review the letterhead and continuation sheets (the paper used for additional pages after the first letterhead page) to adjust the left, right, top, and bottom margins as needed.

In the full block format, all text begins flush with the left margin. This includes the date, address, reference line, salutation, the body of the letter with double spacing for each new paragraph, the complimentary close, and signature line. Tabs are not used as all paragraphs are flush left.

In the modified block format, the date, complimentary close, and signature line are placed just to the right of the middle of the page. An acceptable variation of the modified block allows each new paragraph within the text of the body of the letter to be double-spaced and indented five spaces or about 1/2 inch.

Address. Use commas to separate the parts of an address in narrative form. Exception: Do not place a comma before the ZIP code.

> **The patient's address is 139 Main Street, Ourtown, CA 90299.**

Always use figures (including 1) to refer to house numbers. Do not use commas.

> **1 Eighth Avenue**
> **1408 51st Street**
> **101st Street**
> **14084 Elm Avenue**

Use *No.* or # before an apartment, suite, or room number but not before a house number.

> **1400 Magnolia Avenue, Apt. #148**

Salutation. Greeting line in letters (*Dear...*). Use courtesy titles (*Dr., Ms*, etc.), followed by a colon or a comma, according to letter style and format you use.

NOTE: While salutation lines continue to be the preferred and common practice, it is acceptable to drop them in form letters or in those instances when the appropriate courtesy title is not known, for example, when you cannot determine whether the person is male or female. *To Whom It May Concern* is another alternative in that instance, but it appears to be losing favor.

Copy designation. Notation of those to whom copies of a report or letter are to be distributed. A carbon copy is increasingly known as a courtesy copy. Abbreviated *cc*. A blind copy designation is noted only on the file copy and on the copy to whom it is sent; other recipients' copies do not indicate the blind copy (thus its name). Abbreviated *bc* or *bcc*.

Place copy designations flush left and two line spaces below the end of the report.

> **bc**   **blind copy**
> **bcc** **blind courtesy copy**
> **c**   **copy**
> **cc**   **courtesy copy, carbon copy**
> **pc**   **photocopy**

Envelope preparation. The US Postal Service offers the following guidelines on their website at www.usps.com:

Automated mail processing machines read addresses on mail pieces from the bottom up and will first look for a city, state, and ZIP code. Then the machines look for a delivery address. If the machines can't find either line, then your mail piece could be delayed or misrouted. Any information below the delivery address line (a logo, a slogan, or an attention line) could confuse the machines and misdirect your mail.

Name or attention line	**JANE L MILLER**
Company	**MILLER ASSOCIATES**
Suite or apartment number	**[STE 2006]**
Delivery address	**1960 W CHELSEA AVE STE 2006**
City, state, ZIP code	**ALLENTOWN PA 18104**

- Always put the recipient's address and the postage on the same side of your mail piece.

- On a letter, the address should be parallel to the longest side.

- Use all capital letters.

- No punctuation.

- At least 10-point font.

- One space between city and state.

- Simple fonts and regular (plain) type.

- Left justified.

- Black type on white or light paper.

- No reverse type styles (white printing on a black background).

- If your address appears inside a window, make sure there is at least 1/8-inch clearance around the address. Sometimes parts of the address slip out of view behind the window and mail processing machines can't read the address.

- If you are using address labels, make sure you don't cut off any important information. Also make sure your labels are on straight. Mail processing machines have trouble reading crooked or slanted information.

Email. Email has become an important communication medium.

Security: When email is used for sending and receiving confidential patient information, whether voice or text files, reasonable precautions should be taken to ensure the protection of that information.

Federal privacy and security regulations demand it, and state and local laws may also apply.

Etiquette: Here are some etiquette essentials to help you use email efficiently and effectively.

- Keep your messages short and simple. This is not the place for a novel.

- Do not write your entire message in uppercase. It is equivalent to shouting, and it is not pleasant or easy to read. SEE WHAT I MEAN?

- Go easy on the abbreviations. Unless you can be sure the reader knows all of your abbreviations, the meaning of your message may be lost.

- Use blind cc when sending a mass message. Your recipients will appreciate your respect of their personal email addresses.

- Close your message with your name. Don't assume that the reader will recognize you by your email address.

- Don't send junk, jokes, or chain letters unless you know the reader wants them.

- Don't send unsolicited attachments. When you do send an attachment, explain in your message what the attachment is, and be sure to scan it for viruses before you send it.

- Include only relevant return text. After several exchanges, the email expands to enormous proportions if complete messages are included.

- Use the spellchecker. Misspelled words don't reflect well on the sender and can be annoying to the reader.

- Use a meaningful subject line. This will assist the reader when prioritizing the order of emails to read.

- Don't put anything in an email that you would not put on a postcard. Email is not ordinarily secure.

diagnosis

Abbreviations in diagnoses. Do not use abbreviations for diagnostic terms in document sections designating impression, admission diagnosis, discharge diagnosis, preoperative diagnosis, and postoperative diagnosis. If you cannot determine the meaning of a dictated abbreviation or acronym, transcribe it as dictated, then flag it, requesting that the originator explain the abbreviation or acronym.

> DICTATED
> **Operation: Left BKA.**
>
> TRANSCRIBED
> **OPERATION: Left below-knee amputation.**

While diagnostic terms must not be abbreviated in statements of diagnoses, some descriptive terms relating to the diagnosis may be abbreviated. Use abbreviations for units of measure.

> **Laceration, 5 mm, left abdomen.**

Numbering diagnoses. In section headings, when diagnosis is dictated, it may be changed to the plural form diagnoses if more than one is listed. When only one diagnosis is given, it is preferable not to number it, even if a number is dictated, because the number gives the appearance that there are additional diagnoses. However, if there are several diagnoses it is preferable to number them even if numbers are not dictated.

> **DIAGNOSIS**
> **Appendicitis.**
>
> *preferred to*
>
> **DIAGNOSIS**
> **1. Appendicitis.**

> DICTATED
> **Diagnosis: Appendicitis, history of "cabbage."**

TRANSCRIBED

DIAGNOSIS
1. **Appendicitis.**
2. **History of coronary artery bypass graft (CABG).**

Psychiatric diagnoses. A multiaxial system is often used in diagnosing psychiatric patients. Axis I is for all psychiatric disorders except mood disorders and mental retardation; axis II is for all personality disorders and mental retardation; axis III is for general medical conditions; axis IV, psychosocial and environmental problems; and axis V is an assessment of function, usually using the global assessment of functioning (GAF) scale. The following example demonstrates a typical psychiatric diagnosis along with the applicable diagnostic codes found in the *Diagnostic and Statistical Manual of Mental Disorders, 4th edition* (DSM-IV), which are consistent with ICD-9-CM and ICD-10 codes.

Axis I	296.2	Major depressive disorder, single episode, severe, without psychotic features.
	305.0	Alcohol abuse.
Axis II	301.6	Dependent personality disorder.
Axis III		None.
Axis IV		Threat of job loss.
Axis V		GAF = 3 (current)

"Same." Do not transcribe "same" when dictated for the discharge diagnosis (meaning same as admission diagnosis) or for the postoperative diagnosis (meaning same as preoperative diagnosis). Repeat the diagnosis in full.

DICTATED
ADMISSION DIAGNOSIS: Cholelithiasis.
Discharge diagnosis: Same.

TRANSCRIBED
ADMISSION DIAGNOSIS: Cholelithiasis.
DISCHARGE DIAGNOSIS: Cholelithiasis.

> DICTATED
> **Preoperative diagnosis: uterine fibroid.**
> **Postoperative diagnosis: same.**
>
> TRANSCRIBED
> **PREOPERATIVE DIAGNOSIS: Uterine fibroid.**
> **POSTOPERATIVE DIAGNOSIS: Uterine fibroid.**

Beware of similar incomplete statements within the names of operations, and transcribe them in full.

> DICTATED
> **Preoperative diagnosis: left testicular hernia.**
>
> TRANSCRIBED
> **PREOPERATIVE DIAGNOSIS: Left testicular hernia.**
>
> DICTATED
> **Operation performed: repair of same.**
>
> TRANSCRIBED
> **OPERATION PERFORMED: Repair of left testicular hernia.**

Differential diagnosis. When a patient presents with a group of symptoms and the diagnosis is unclear, the clinician may refer in the medical report to the differential diagnosis in order to compare and contrast the clinical findings of each. Although it consists of two or more possible diagnoses, the term differential diagnosis itself is singular and always takes a singular verb.

> **The differential diagnosis was . . .**

discharge summary

The report that recapitulates the reason for hospitalization, the significant findings, the procedures performed and treatment rendered, the condition of the patient on discharge, and the discharge plan is commonly known as the "discharge summary" or "clinical summary."

Typical content headings in a discharge summary include

chief complaint
admitting diagnosis
history of present illness
pertinent past history (past medical history)
physical examination on discharge
laboratory findings
hospital course
condition on discharge
discharge diagnoses (or final diagnoses)
disposition
prognosis
discharge instructions and medications
followup plans

formats

While various institutional formats are acceptable, standardized formats for many report types have been developed by the Healthcare Informatics committee of ASTM in a standard called E2184, Standard Specification for Healthcare Document Formats, which specifies the requirements for the sections and subsections, and their arrangement, in an individual's healthcare documents. Some of the formatting suggestions in this book—in particular H&Ps and similar reports—are consistent with those published in the ASTM standard.

Block format is preferred (all lines flush left) for all reports, as well as for correspondence, but institutional and client preferences may vary and should prevail.

Margins. Leave half-inch to one-inch margins, top and bottom, left and right.

Ragged-right margins are preferred over right-justified margins, with all lines flush left (block format).

To enhance readability, avoid end-of-line hyphenation except for terms with pre-existing hyphens.

Paragraphs. Use paragraphs to separate narrative blocks within sections. In general, start new paragraphs as dictated except when such paragraphing is excessive (some originators start a new paragraph with every sentence or two) or inadequate (some originators dictate an entire lengthy report in one paragraph).

Section and subsection headings. Title reports and report sections as dictated, unless you are following a standardized format. Institutional and client preferences should prevail.

Use all capitals for major section headings. Use initial capitals for subsection headings.

Avoid underlining because it diminishes readability.

List chief complaint, diagnoses, preoperative diagnoses, postoperative diagnoses, names of operations, and similar entries vertically. If the originator numbers some but not all items, be consistent and number all or none. When a single diagnosis is referred to as "number one," it is better to delete the number so that the reader is not led to believe that additional entries are missing.

Obvious headings that are not dictated may be inserted, but this is not required. If the originator moves in and out of sections, insert the information into the appropriate sections. (Headings may be omitted where appropriate.)

Double-space between major sections of reports.

List subsection headings vertically to assist the reader in identifying particular subsections.

Do not use abbreviations or brief forms in headings except for such widely used and readily recognizable abbreviations as HEENT, if dictated.

Place the content on the next line following the section or subsection heading, if possible. The ASTM "Formats" standard calls for an extra line space between subheadings, as in the following example.

> **HEENT**
> **Within normal limits.**
>
> **Thorax and Lungs**
> **No rales or rhonchi.**
>
> **Cardiovascular**
> **No murmurs.**

When the information following the section or subsection heading continues on the same line, use a colon (not a hyphen or a dash) after each heading.

> **HEENT: Within normal limits.**
> **THORAX AND LUNGS: No rales or rhonchi.**
> **CARDIOVASCULAR: No murmurs.**

Capitalize the word following the heading, whether or not a colon follows the heading. Exception: When quantity and unit of measure immediately follow a heading, such as estimated blood loss, use numerals.

> **LUNGS: Within normal limits.**
> **ESTIMATED BLOOD LOSS: 10 mL.**

End each entry with a period unless it is a date or the name of a person.

> **ANESTHESIOLOGIST: Sharon Smith, MD**
> **ANESTHESIA: General.**

Signature block. Enter the signature block four lines below the final line of text, flush left. Use the originator's full name. If a title is given, place it directly below the originator's name; use initial capitals, unless institutional style calls for all caps. Note: Signature lines are often preformatted; in that case, leave as formatted.

> **Ruth T. Gross, MD**
> **Chief of Pediatrics**

Initials of originator and transcriptionist at end of transcript. It is common practice to include originator and transcriptionist initials at the end of each report. When used, enter the initials flush left two lines below last line of text. Use either all capitals or all lowercase letters for both sets of initials, with a colon or virgule between them. Do not use periods.

Do not include academic degrees, professional credentials, or titles.

> **RH:ST** *or* **rh:st**
> **RH/ST** *or* **rh/st**

Some facilities may choose to identify the originators and MTs by other identifiers, such as a number or a number-letter combination, and system-generated reports may enter these identifiers automatically along with date, time, and place stamps.

> DICTATED
> **D283, 02/02/02, 2:35 p.m., Indianapolis, IN**
>
> TRANSCRIBED
> **T149, 02/02/02, 11:40 p.m., LaFayette, IN**

Time and date stamp. For the sake of an audit trail, it is common practice to include the date and time of dictation and transcription at the end of each report. Enter the date and time flush left below the initials of the originator and transcriptionist. Use colons for the time unless military time is the preferred format.

NOTE: Identification of the place of dictation and transcription may be required as well.

> **D: 02/02/02, 11:40 p.m., LaFayette, IN**
> **T: 2/3/02, 8:45 a.m., Springfield, MO**

Continuation pages. When a transcript is longer than one page, enter continued at the bottom of each printed page prior to the last, and repeat the patient's name and medical record number, the page number, the type and date of report on each continuation page. Additional identifying data may be noted, according to the employer's or client's preference.

Do not carry a single line of a report onto a continuation page. Do not allow a continuation page to include only the signature block and the data following it.

When the printing is done by someone other than the medical transcriptionist, or when it is programmed into the system, these guidelines should still be followed.

NOTE: The guidelines above cannot be applied in electronic environments where formatting is automatically generated by the technology. In those instances, the MT should follow facility guidelines for allowing text to wrap and flow from start to finish without formatting for page breaks.

history and physical examination

Abbreviation: *H&P* (no spaces, no periods). Typical major content headings in a history and physical, taken from ASTM's E2184, Standard Specification for Healthcare Document Formats, include the following:

CHIEF COMPLAINT
HISTORY OF PRESENT ILLNESS
PAST HISTORY
ALLERGIES
CURRENT MEDICATIONS
REVIEW OF SYSTEMS
PHYSICAL EXAMINATION
MENTAL STATUS EXAMINATION
DIAGNOSTIC STUDIES
DIAGNOSIS
ORDERS

operative report

Typical content headings in an operative report include:

PREOPERATIVE DIAGNOSIS
POSTOPERATIVE DIAGNOSIS
REASON FOR OPERATION *or* **INDICATIONS**
OPERATION PERFORMED *or* **NAME OF OPERATION**
SURGEON
ASSISTANTS
ANESTHESIOLOGIST
ANESTHESIA
INDICATIONS FOR PROCEDURE
FINDINGS
PROCEDURE OR TECHNIQUE
COMPLICATIONS
TOURNIQUET TIME
HARDWARE
DRAINS
SPECIMENS
ESTIMATED BLOOD LOSS

> **INSTRUMENT AND SPONGE COUNTS**
> **DISPOSITION OF PATIENT**
> **FOLLOWUP**

progress note   An interim note in a patient's medical record, made by medical staff and other authorized personnel.

SOAP note   One format used for patient care documentation, especially in problem-oriented medical records. The acronym SOAP stands for:

S   subjective (patient's descriptions)

O   objective (clinician's observations)

A   assessment (clinician's interpretations)

P   plan (clinician's treatment plan)

type style   **Regular type.** Also known as plain type, regular type is preferred throughout medical transcription, with just a few exceptions when bold type or italics may be preferred or required for emphasis or to conform to a facility's model or a client's personal style.

Bold type. In general, avoid bold type in medical transcription. A common exception is the use of bold type to designate a patient's allergies, although regular type is also acceptable.

> **ALLERGIES: PENICILLIN.**

NOTE: ASTM's E2184, Standard Specification for Healthcare Document Formats, calls for all major headings in the report as well as allergies (the heading and the substance to which the individual is allergic) to be expressed in all capital letters but with regular type (not bold).

Italics. Use regular type, not italics, for English and medical terms as well as for foreign words and phrases that are commonly used in the English language and in medical reports.

bruit
cul-de-sac
en masse
in toto
peau d'orange
poudrage

Use regular type, as well, in the following instances even though italics may be called for in manuscript preparation:

abbreviations: AFO

arbitrary designations: patient B

chemical elements: boron

Latin names of genera and species: Clostridium difficile

letters indicating shape: T-bar

names of foreign institutions and organizations

NOTE: Italics and other attributes such as bolding may be lost in electronic transmission of reports.

The Final Word

For samples of each of the document types defined above, see Appendix A. In addition, keep in mind that more report samples can be found in the appendices of each *Stedman's Word Book* series text by specialty. When learning the pause and flow of narrative in the medical record, it is a good idea to read and study sample reports to become more familiar with report organization and formatting. Always balance clarity of communication with any decision to alter a formatting recommendation outlined here.

Test Your Knowledge

Correct the errors in each of the sentences below.

1. DIAGNOSIS
   1. Urinary tract infection.

2. ESTIMATED BLOOD LOSS: Ten milliliters.

3. Lungs: clear to auscultation and percussion.

4. ADMITTING DIAGNOSIS
   1. Hypertension, uncontrolled.
   2. Extreme fatigue.

5. PREOPERATIVE DIAGNOSIS
   Ureterolithiasis.

   POSTOPERATIVE DIAGNOSIS
   Same.

6. She lives at 555 Oak Street, Smallville, FL, 59999.

7. DIAGNOSES
   Coronary artery disease.

8. OPERATION
   CABG.

9. HEART: regular rate and rhythm.

10. Stool culture was positive for *E. coli*.

Test Your Knowledge

Answers

---

1. DIAGNOSIS
Urinary tract infection.

---

2. ESTIMATED BLOOD LOSS: 10 mL.

---

3. Lungs: Clear to auscultation and percussion.

---

4. ADMITTING DIAGNOSES
1. Hypertension, uncontrolled.
2. Extreme fatigue.

---

5. PREOPERATIVE DIAGNOSIS
Ureterolithiasis.

POSTOPERATIVE DIAGNOSIS
Ureterolithiasis.

---

6. She lives at 555 Oak Street, Smallville, FL 59999.

---

7. DIAGNOSIS
Coronary artery disease.

---

8. OPERATION
Coronary artery bypass graft.

---

9. HEART: Regular rate and rhythm.

---

10. Stool culture was positive for E. coli.

The Medical Record: Security, Access & Modification

If transcriptionists were only required to "type what they hear" and apply the standards as outlined throughout this book, the role would be a relatively straightforward and unencumbered one. There are some in healthcare who advocate this kind of restricted role for documentation specialists, embracing a "verbatim" transcription policy that limits the MT to transcribing only what is dictated, whether right or wrong, and flagging discrepancies for review by the dictator. In most environments, however, there is the expectation that the MT will be actively engaged in the story-telling of the patient encounter, noting discrepancies in grammar, style, and clinical information, and correcting those discrepancies that fall within the scope of the MTs knowledge and informed judgment. Certainly, routing discrepancies back to the dictator that could have been reasonably corrected by the transcriptionist has a direct impact on turn-around time and reimbursement. Such a restrictive policy for editing and correction can be costly to the facility and burdensome to the medical records department who has to facilitate those corrections. A skilled, engaged MT partners with the physician to ensure an accurate, timely, and secure record.

This chapter will provide an overview of those standards in the BOS that address management and modification of the medical record and will answer many of the questions that plague a new MT: *What do you do when you can't understand what is being dictated? Skip it? Guess? When am I allowed to edit what is dictated, especially when I know that what is being dictated is wrong?* There are guidelines provided here for managing the records you will be entrusted with, including the important subjects of HIPAA privacy, confidentiality, record access, and modifying or changing a patient record. In addition those provided below, make sure to read Appendix C: *Modifying the Patient Record: Corrections, Revisions, Additions, and Addenda.*

Going Deeper

On the subject of HIPAA, which has changed policies and procedures throughout healthcare where privacy and security of patient health information are concerned, the *BOS* provides only definition and overview of this important subject. Before entering the workforce, you will need to be well informed about the expectations related to compliance that are placed on medical transcriptionists, particularly those who work from home. To that end, AAMT has prepared an extensive packet of information designed to assist MTs in understanding and ensuring at-home HIPAA compliance. This document, *HIPAA for MTs,* is free to AAMT members, including AAMT student members, and available for purchase by nonmembers at the AAMT website (www.aamt.org).

Rules & Exceptions

audit trails   Also known as documentation trails, audit trails contribute to risk management. An audit trail is simply a careful sequential record of actions and conversations on a particular matter. This type of record is recommended for any event considered legally sensitive, including circumstances where medical transcriptionists are advised or directed to act contrary to usual practices or legal directives.

confidentiality Patients have a legal and ethical right to the reasonable expectation that their private information will not be disclosed except for the purposes for which it was provided (such as receiving healthcare services). Medical transcriptionists share with other healthcare personnel the responsibility to respect the confidentiality of medical records. Federal and state laws govern the extent of confidentiality required and the exceptions under which disclosure can be made.

Confidentiality is sometimes confused with two related but different concepts: privacy and privilege. Privacy means an individual's right to be left alone and/or to decide what to share with others. Privacy may, for example, affect whether gratuitous, irrelevant, and personal information is even included in a record. Privilege means the legal protection against being forced to violate confidentiality in a legal proceeding, such as by disclosing confidential records.

HIPAA privacy rule. The Health Insurance Portability and Accountability Act of 1996 (HIPAA) includes regulations related to the privacy of health information. The HIPAA privacy rule requires healthcare providers and others who maintain health information to put in place measures to guard the privacy and confidentiality of patient information. Before HIPAA, patient privacy was only sporadically protected by various laws—never so dramatically as it is by the HIPAA statute and its accompanying regulations. The text of the rule, published in the Federal Register on December 28, 2000, can be found on the Administrative Simplification website of the US Department of Health and Human Services: http://aspe.hhs.gov/admnsimp.

Some states may have more stringent privacy requirements than those contained in the HIPAA privacy rule. It behooves every medical transcription business owner to understand the applicable state laws and make a determination as to which is more stringent, and the business owner should seek the advice of an attorney in this regard.

Protecting patient information. The HIPAA privacy rule regulates the use and disclosure of specifically identifiable health information regarding the physical or mental health or condition of an individual. The rule applies directly to those entities that typically generate individually identifiable patient health information and therefore have primary responsibility for maintaining the privacy and confidentiality of such information. As a general matter, a so-called "covered entity" may use or disclose protected health information only with an individual's written consent or authorization. However, health information can be disclosed without consent or authorization for certain purposes, such as research and public health, if specified conditions are met. Covered entities also must comply with a host of administrative requirements intended to protect patient privacy.

The privacy rule also applies indirectly to business associates of covered entities. Medical transcriptionists who contract directly with healthcare providers fall into this category. The privacy rule requires covered entities to enter into a written agreement with each business associate—known as a business associate agreement. Significantly, the business associate may not use or disclose the protected health information other than as permitted or required by the business associate agreement or as required by law. Subcontractors must agree to essentially the same conditions and restrictions as business associates with respect to the use and disclosure of protected health information.

Within the body of the medical report, care should be taken to avoid mentioning personally identifying information. For example, it is common practice for a medical transcriptionist to replace the dictated patient's name with simply "the patient" or perhaps, "the above-named patient." What follows is a list of identifiers that are best avoided in medical reports, whether in reference to a patient or to a patient's relatives, employers, or household members.

name
address
dates (e.g., date of birth, admission and discharge dates)
telephone and fax numbers
email addresses
Social Security numbers
medical record numbers

> health plan beneficiary numbers
> account numbers
> certificate/license numbers
> vehicle identifiers, including license plate numbers
> device identifiers and serial numbers
> Web Universal Resource Locators (URL)
> Internet protocol (IP) address numbers
> biometric identifiers (e.g., finger and voice prints)
> full-face photographic images and any comparable images
> any other unique identifying number, characteristic, or code

NOTE: The HIPAA privacy rule makes clear provisions for "de-identifying" a record so that it is no longer considered protected health information. While the above list of identifiers is similar to the list found in the privacy rule, if your intention is to actually de-identify the record you will need to refer to the rule itself—as well as legal counsel—for specific guidelines.

Retention of records. For the medical transcriptionist, discussions about retaining healthcare records generally apply to patient logs, dictated tapes or digital voice files, and transcribed reports (whether print or electronic). AAMT recommends that independent MTs and MT businesses retain such information only as long as is absolutely necessary to conduct business, that is, no longer than necessary for verification, distribution, and billing purposes. This opinion is shared by the authors of ASTM's E1 902, Standard Guide for Management of the Confidentiality and Security of Dictation, Transcription, and Transcribed Health Records.

date dictated, date transcribed

These dates should be recorded to monitor dictation and transcription patterns as well as to provide documentation of when the work (dictation or transcription) was done. Some dictation and transcription systems are specially designed to automatically record these dates.

Healthcare reports are, among other things, legal documents. As part of risk management, dictation and transcription dates should be entered accurately and should not be altered.

Capitalize D and T and follow each by a colon and appropriate date, using numerals separated by virgules or hyphens.

Some facilities prefer to use six-digit dates and others, eight-digit. All these styles are acceptable.

> **D: 4/18/00**
> **T: 4/19/00**
>
> **D: 04-18-00**
> **T: 04-19-00**
>
> **D: 04/18/2000**
> **T: 04/19/2000**

NOTE: ASTM's E2184, Standard Specification for Healthcare Document Formats calls for identification of the place of dictation as well.

dictated but not read

Some originators or transcription supervisors direct that the statement "dictated but not read" (or a similar phrase such as "transcribed but not read" or "signed but not read") be entered at the end of a report in an attempt to waive the originator's responsibility to review the report and confirm its accuracy.

It is not appropriate for an MT to enter this statement because the MT can verify only that the report was transcribed; only the originator can verify that it was not read (and the latter is a fact that may change later). In addition, not reading records is a practice MTs should not encourage.

AAMT advises against the use of such phrases. A patient's report is authenticated when it is signed; the signature indicates that the report is accurate in the eyes of the authenticator, usually the report's originator. Medical transcriptionists must make every effort to be sure the report is transcribed accurately, but the final responsibility and authority lie with the originator. If the MT is required to enter this statement, it is advisable to get the directive in writing, to document one's objections to it, and to retain that documentation should it be necessary to defend the action in the future.

dictation problems

A variety of dictation problems may occur, and medical transcriptionists being alert to them is a form of risk management. Watch for and correct obvious errors in dictation, including grammar, spelling, terminology, and style. When uncertain, draw suspected errors to the attention of the originator and/or supervisor. When the change would be significant, particularly if it would influence medical meaning, leave a blank and flag it.

Blank. Leave a blank when a dictated term, phrase, or abbreviation is unintelligible (whether due to equipment problems or mispronunciation) or cannot be confirmed through reasonable research; flag the report, briefly explaining why you left a blank, noting what the dictation sounds like, and asking for feedback for future reference.

Never "close up" the space where the unintelligible word, phrase, or sentence belongs, making it appear that a transcript is complete. Likewise, do not transcribe the questionable dictation, adding [sic] to indicate it is transcribed verbatim.

When the transcriptionist cannot determine how to edit the incorrect dictation properly, sometimes the best choice is to leave a blank and flag it. Appropriate use of blanks should prompt careful followup and contribute to patient care and risk management.

Flag. A flag is a notation by the medical transcriptionist to the originator of a report, drawing attention to missing data, unclear dictation, errors in dictation, inconsistent dictation, equipment problems, potentially inflammatory remarks, etc. Flags contribute to risk management.

When flagging a printed report, cite the page, section, and line number. If the word or phrase is unfamiliar, note what it sounds like. If the term is inconsistent, briefly state why, e.g., "A left below-knee amputation is later referred to as right BK amputation. Which is correct?" Similarly, flag medical inconsistencies you are unsure of, in order to permit review by the report's originator to assure accuracy. Many systems now have methods in place to provide an "electronic flag," which should be noted as above, using the instructions for that particular system.

Inconsistencies in dictation. A medical transcriptionist who identifies an inconsistency in dictation should resolve it if this can be done with competence and confidence. If the discrepancy cannot be resolved with certainty, the report should be flagged and brought to the attention of the supervisor or the report's originator for resolution.

> **This 45-year-old male is status post hysterectomy. (Either the patient is not male or he is status post another type of surgery.)**

editing

Verbatim transcription of dictation is seldom possible. MTs should prepare reports that are as correct, clear, consistent, and complete as can be reasonably expected, without imposing their personal style on those reports. Tools for editing include dictionaries, wordbooks, stylebooks, textbooks, grammar software, other teaching materials, experts, and experience.

> DICTATED
> **The patient developed a puffy right eye that was felt to be secondary to an insect bite by the ophthalmologist.**
>
> TRANSCRIBED
> **The patient developed a puffy right eye; this was felt by the ophthalmologist to be secondary to an insect bite.**
>
> DICTATED
> **CAT scan showed there was nothing in the brain but sinusitis.**
>
> TRANSCRIBED
> **CAT scan of the brain showed only sinusitis.**

Editing is inappropriate in medical transcription when it alters information without the editor's being certain of the appropriateness or accuracy of the change, when it second-guesses the originator, when it deletes appropriate and/or essential information, and when it tampers with the originator's style.

Edit grammar, punctuation, spelling, and similar dictation errors as necessary to achieve clear communication. Likewise, edit slang words and phrases, incorrect terms, incomplete phrases, English or medical inconsistencies, and inaccurate phrasing of laboratory data.

DICTATED
temp

TRANSCRIBED
temperature

DICTATED
Operation: Teflon tube.

TRANSCRIBED
Operation: Teflon tube insertion.

When transcribing dictation by those who speak English as a second language, edit obvious errors, following the general guidelines for editing. It is not necessary or recommended that such dictation be rewritten; rather, the physician's basic style should be retained.

Transcription businesses and departments should establish clear policies and instructions on how to deal with inappropriate language or inflammatory remarks in dictation. Medical transcriptionists should check with their supervisors to determine the rules for editing or omitting such language and remarks from transcription.

Institutional policy and originator preference are major factors in decisions to edit. To the extent that editing is acceptable in your setting and to the originator, the following guidelines for editing are recommended.

Clarifying content. Refer to the patient's record to clarify or correct content in dictation. If the record is not available, draw attention to errors or potentially confusing entries for which you do not have sufficient information to make corrections.

Leaving blanks. Leave a blank space in a report rather than guessing what was meant or transcribing unclear or obviously incorrect dictation. Flag the report to draw attention to the blank.

Flagging reports. When flagging a report to draw attention to unclear or incorrect dictation, cite the page, section, and line number, tagging the error on paper or electronically. If the word or phrase is unfamiliar, note what it sounds like. If the term is inconsistent, briefly state why, e.g., "A left below-knee amputation is later referred to as right BK amputation. Which is correct?"

Similarly, draw attention to medical inconsistencies you have corrected, in order to encourage the originator's review to assure accuracy.

Negative findings. Never delete negative or normal findings if dictated. To do so is altering the dictation as well as the medical record. See: negative findings.

Speech recognition and editing. The computerized translation by a speech recognition engine of dictated material results in text that usually needs considerable editing. This is sometimes done by the originator but more often by a person with the medical knowledge and language skills of a medical transcriptionist, who ideally will review the text while listening to the originator's voice file, checking for errors and inconsistencies. The same editing guidelines that apply to medical transcription apply to editing the text resulting from speech-recognized dictation.

HIPAA
The Health Insurance Portability and Accountability Act of 1996 is legislation created to save costs by simplifying the administration of health care. Administered by the US Department of Health and Human Services, HIPAA includes regulations related to healthcare transactions and code sets, privacy of health information, security of information, and the establishment of national identifiers for providers and employers.

JCAHO
Abbreviation for Joint Commission on Accreditation of Healthcare Organizations, an independent, not-for-profit organization that develops organizational standards, awards accreditation decisions, and provides education and consultation to healthcare organizations.

originator's style
The transcriptionist is responsible for retaining the originator's style when translating the spoken word to text. Yet, the MT must also edit to assure the record's completeness, correctness, coherence, clarity, and read-

20|6

ability. There is a fine line between appropriate editing, which the transcriptionist must do, and tampering, which the transcriptionist must diligently avoid.

proofreading   Proofread all reports. MTs should proofread reports while transcribing, after completing transcription, and (when there is access to the printed copy) after printing the report.

For many MTs, there is no access to the printed report because it is transmitted electronically and/or printed remotely. In this circumstance, MTs must use their on-screen proofreading skills both during and after completion of the transcript. Spellcheckers and grammar checkers are supplements to, not replacements for, proofreading. Some transcription departments and businesses designate specific personnel as proofreaders. This does not release MTs from the responsibility to proofread their own work.

quality assurance   Quality assurance (QA) for medical transcription contributes to risk management. A standard has been developed by ASTM's Healthcare Informatics committee called E2117, Standard Guide for Identification and Establishment of a Quality Assurance Program for Medical Transcription. This standard clearly defines the roles of the medical transcriptionist, the QA reviewer, the management staff, as well as the originator of the medical report.

release of information   Release of protected health information involves both legal requirements and professional responsibility. MTs should not release information except as authorized by institutional policies and procedures, and consistent with the law. The patient's rights to personal and informational privacy and confidentiality must be respected. At the same time, courts and others may have legitimate rights to health information that MTs must recognize.

The HIPAA privacy regulations use the term "disclosure" for what has historically been known as release of information. A separate consent from the patient may be required for each disclosure, and audit trails are required for each disclosure made. Care should be taken to assure that all disclosures are made in accordance with current laws and rules.

risk management

Healthcare institution activities that identify, evaluate, reduce, and prevent the risk of injury and loss to patients, visitors, staff, and the institution itself.

Medical transcriptionists play an important role in risk management through their commitment to quality in medical transcription and through their alertness to dictated information that indicates potential risk to the patient or the institution, including its personnel. When encountered, such information should be brought to the attention of the appropriate institutional personnel, as identified in the institution's program policies.

Cross-references below address some of the topics that relate medical transcription to risk management.

security

Security precautions must be taken to protect health information in the electronic systems on which that information is stored and by which it is transferred. The voluntary standard published by ASTM International, E1902, *Standard Guide for Management of the Confidentiality and Security of Dictation, Transcription, and Transcribed Health Records,* takes the reader through the entire dictation and transcription process and points out areas where the record must be made secure. In addition, AAMT has published a document titled *HIPAA for MTs: Considerations for the Medical Transcriptionist as Business Associate,* which contains specific advice concerning the HIPAA privacy rule as well as guidance on protecting the security of healthcare documentation.

verbatim transcription

Most dictation cannot be transcribed verbatim if it is to be complete, comprehensible, and consistent, since few people speak in a manner that allows conversion into printed form without at least minor editing.

Nevertheless, medical transcriptionists may be required to transcribe some or all reports verbatim. Unless the dictation is perfect (which is unlikely), the MT should retain some evidence of the directive. If the facility guidelines allow, the transcriptionist may choose to enter the statement "transcribed verbatim" at the end of the report, in order to defend the transcript in the future if necessary.

The Final Word

A patient's record is an important story, one that needs to accurately reflect the exchange of information that occurred between the provider and the patient during that encounter. Preserving the tone and scope of that encounter while ensuring the accuracy of the data being captured is critical to creating a long-term care record that is historically and clinically meaningful. The *art* of managing information that ensures this outcome falls within the skill set of the transcriptionist. Honoring a physician's dictation style, recognizing error or inconsistency in the record, correcting errors appropriately, refraining from correcting or altering what cannot be confirmed, protecting the integrity of the patient encounter, and ensuring the confidentiality of the record that results are *at the heart* of what you as a medical transcriptionist will be engaged in every day. This will require a dedication to detail and a commitment to vigilance that goes beyond simple interpretation of medical terminology.

Test Your Knowledge

Answer the scenario questions below to check your understanding of the material covered in this chapter.

1. The physician accidentally dictates, "Sodium 4.2 and potassium 141." What do you do?

2. The physician dictates the patient's home address and telephone number in the body of the report. What should you do?

3. You are an independent contractor and your physician client has asked you to keep copies of all transcribed records for the purposes of backup. How do you respond?

4. The physician dictates from his cell phone, and as a result, a few words are garbled and indecipherable in his dictation. What do you do?

5. In a recent wrongful death court case, where a patient died while waiting for critically needed surgery to be scheduled, the transcriptionist was blamed for the delay in scheduling because of an alleged delay in transcribing the consultation report needed by the insurance company to approve the surgery. The transcriptionist testified that she transcribed the patient's consultation report within 24 hours and that the delay was not her fault. How would date/time stamping have supported the transcriptionist's claim?

Test Your Knowledge

Answers

1. Unless you are working in a verbatim environment where you are not allowed to edit the dictation, you should correct this discrepancy without flagging or alerting the dictator. This is a common mistake made by providers who are dictating quickly, and even a relatively new transcriptionist should recognize the transposition of two laboratory values that are commonly dictated together. Correct transcription: *Sodium 141 and potassium 4.2.*

2. Check with your supervisor (or client if you are self-employed) about facility policy for inclusion of protected health information (PHI) in the body of patient reports. If facility policy restricts this inclusion, remove this information, and flag the deletion to the attention of the physician.

3. Educate your client about the restrictions imposed by HIPAA for retention of records by a business associate. HIPAA restricts contact to patient records by a business associate to whatever is "minimally necessary" for provision of services. Once you have provided those services as an MT, you no longer have a legal right to have access to those records, and your physician client needs to make other arrangements for long-term backup of his/her patient records.

4. Leave a blank in the appropriate place, flag the dictation per your facility's designated procedures for flagging, and direct the report back to the dictating physician for revision.

5. For audit trail purposes, the date and time stamp clearly document when the report was dictated and when it was transcribed. For just such reasons as were present in this case, date and time stamps help to provide chronology where patient care documentation is concerned. Such a date and time stamp on the consultation report in question would have supported the transcriptionist's claim that the report was transcribed within the expected time frame.

NOTE: There are no CD exercises for this chapter.